Chemical Ranking and Scoring
Guidelines for Relative Assessments of Chemicals

Other titles from the Society of Environmental Toxicology and Chemistry (SETAC):

Chemically Induced Alterations in Functional Development and Reproduction of Fishes
R.M. Rolland, M. Gilbertson, R.E. Peterson, editors

Atmospheric Deposition of Contaminants to the Great Lakes and Coastal Waters
J.E. Baker, editor

Ecological Risk Assessment of Contaminated Sediments
C.G. Ingersoll, T. Dillon, G.R. Biddinger, editors

Reassessment of Metals Criteria for Aquatic Life Protection:
Priorities for Research and Implementation
H.L. Bergman and E.J. Dorward-King, editors

Whole Effluent Toxicity Testing:
An Evaluation of Methods and Prediction of Receiving System Impacts
D.R. Grothe, K.L. Dickson, D.K. Reed-Judkins, editors

The Multi-Media Fate Model:
A Vital Tool for Predicting the Fate of Chemicals
C.E. Cowan, D. Mackay, T.C.J. Feijtel, D. Van de Meent, A. DiGuardo,
J. Davies, N. Mackay, editors

Aquatic Dialogue Group: Pesticide Risk Assessment and Mitigation
J.L. Baker, A.C. Barefoot, L.E. Beasley, L. Burns, P. Caulkins, J. Clark,
R.L. Feulner, J.P. Giesy, R.L. Graney, R. Griggs, H. Jacoby, D. Laskowski,
A. Maciorowski, E. Mihaich, H. Nelson, R. Parrish, R.E. Siefert, K.R. Solomon,
W. van der Schalie, editors

For information about additional titles or about SETAC's international journal,
Environmental Toxicology and Chemistry,
contact the SETAC Office, 1010 N. 12th Avenue, Pensacola, Florida, USA 32501-3370
T 850 469 1500   F 850 469 9778   E setac@setac.org   http://www.setac.org

Chemical Ranking and Scoring
Guidelines for Relative Assessments of Chemicals

Edited by

Mary B. Swanson, M.S.
University of Tennessee

Adam C. Socha, M.Sc.
Ontario Ministry of Environment and Energy

Proceedings of the Pellston Workshop on Chemical Ranking and Scoring
12–16 February 1995
Sandestin, Florida

SETAC Special Publications Series

Current Series Editor
C.G. Ingersoll, Ph. D.
U.S. Geological Survey, Midwest Science Center

Past Series Editors
T.W. La Point, Ph.D.
The Institute of Wildlife and Environmental Toxicology, Clemson University

B.T. Walton, Ph.D.
U.S. Office of Science and Technology Policy, Executive Office of the President

C.H. Ward, Ph.D.
Department of Environmental Sciences and Engineering, Rice University

Publication sponsored by the Society of Environmental Toxicology and Chemistry
(SETAC) and the SETAC Foundation for Environmental Education

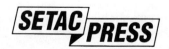

Cover by Michael Kenney Graphic Design and Advertising
Typesetting by Wordsmiths Unlimited

Library of Congress Cataloging-in-Publication Data

Pellston Workshop on Chemical Ranking & Scoring (1995 : Sandestin, Fla.)
  Chemical ranking and scoring : guidelines for relative assessments of chemicals : proceedings of the Pellston Workshop on Chemical Ranking & Scoring, 12-16 February 1995, Sandestin, Florida / edited by Mary B. Swanson, Adam C. Socha.
      p. cm. -- (SETAC special publications series)
  Publication sponsored by the Society of Environmental Toxicology and Chemistry (SETAC) and the SETAC Foundation for Environmental Education.
  Includes bibliographical references and index.
  ISBN 1-880611-12-0
  1. Health risk assessment--Methodology--Congresses. 2. Environmental toxicology--Congresses. I. Swanson, Mary B. (Mary Beth), 1962. II. Socha, Adam C. (Adam Charles), 1961– III. SETAC (Society). IV. SETAC Foundation for Environmental Education. V. Title. VI. Series.
RA566.27.P45 1995
615.9'02--DC21   97-29783
                                                                                                        CIP

Information in this book was obtained from individual experts and highly regarded sources. It is the publisher's intent to print accurate and reliable information, and numerous references are cited; however, the authors, editors, and publisher cannot be responsible for the validity of all information presented here or for the consequences of its use. Information contained herein does not necessarily reflect the policy or views of the Society of Environmental Toxicology and Chemistry (SETAC) or the SETAC Foundation for Environmental Education.

International Standard Book Number 1-880611-12-0
Printed in the United States of America
04 03 02 01 00 99 98 97   10 9 8 7 6 5 4 3 2 1

∞ The paper used in this publication meets the minimum requirements of the American National Standard for Information Sciences—Permanence of Paper for Printed Library Materials, ANSI Z39.48-1984.

Reference Listing: Swanson MB, Socha AC, editors. 1997. Chemical ranking and scoring: guidelines for relative assessments of chemicals. Proceedings of the Pellston Workshop on Chemical Ranking and Scoring; 12–16 February 1995; Sandestin FL. Published by the Society of Environmental Toxicology and Chemistry (SETAC), Pensacola, Florida, USA. 186 p.

The SETAC Special Publications Series

The SETAC Special Publications Series was established by the Society of Environmental Toxicology and Chemistry (SETAC) to provide in-depth reviews and critical appraisals on scientific subjects relevant to understanding the impacts of chemicals and technology on the environment. The series consists of single- and multiple-authored or edited books on topics reviewed and recommended by the SETAC Board of Directors for their importance, timeliness, and contribution to multidisciplinary approaches to solving environmental problems. The diversity and breadth of subjects covered in the series reflect the wide range of disciplines encompassed by environmental toxicology, environmental chemistry, and hazard and risk assessment. Despite this diversity, the goals of these volumes are similar; they are to present the reader with authoritative coverage of the literature, as well as paradigms, methodologies and controversies, research needs, and new developments specific to the featured topics. All books in the series are peer reviewed for SETAC by acknowledged experts.

The SETAC Special Publications are useful to environmental scientists in research, research management, chemical manufacturing, regulation, and education, as well as to students considering careers in these areas. The series provides information for keeping abreast of recent developments in familiar subject areas and for rapid introduction to principles and approaches in new subject areas.

Chemical Ranking and Scoring: Guidelines for Relative Assessments of Chemicals presents the collected papers stemming from a SETAC-sponsored Pellston Workshop on Chemical Ranking and Scoring held in Sandestin, Florida, 12–16 February 1995. The workshop focused on developing a framework and guidance for developing and using chemical ranking and scoring.

Contents

Chapter 1: Framework for Chemical Ranking and Scoring Systems 1
*Gary Davis (chapter editor), Dan Fort, Bjørn Hansen, Fran Irwin,
Baxter Jones, Sheila Jones, Adam Socha, Robert Wilson, Bill Haaf,
George Gray, Bill Hoffman*

Chapter 2: Measures of Exposure 31
*Mary Swanson (chapter editor), Bob Boethling, John Evans,
John Geisy, Jim Gillett, Phil Howard, David Jeffrey, Jay Jon,
Preben Kristensen, Robert Larson, Yong-Hwa Kim*

Chapter 3: Human Health Effects 61
*Gary Hurlburt (chapter editor), Rolf Bretz, Emma Lou George,
Rolf Hartung, Ray Kent, Lynne Fahey McGrath, Ron Newhook,
Mike Stevens, Brad Strohm, Pauline Wagner*

Chapter 4: Ecological Effects 89
*Rich Kimerle (chapter editor), Larry Barnthouse, Richard Brown,
Bernard Conilh de Beyssac, Mike Gilbertson, Kathy Monk,
Heinz-Jochen Poremski, Richard Purdy, Kevin Reinert,
Rosalind Rolland, Maurice Zeeman*

Chapter 5: Other Chemical Characteristics 113
*Allan A. Jensen and John Walker (chapter editors), Franz Fiala,
Karim Ahmed, Mark Ralston, Robert Ross, Friedrich Schmidt-Bleek,
Duane Tolle*

List of Figures

List of Tables

Foreword

This workshop was a continuation of a series of successful workshops called the "Pellston Workshop Series." Since 1977, twenty-seven workshops have been held at Pellston and several other locations to evaluate current and prospective environmental issues. Each has focused on a relevant environmental topic, and the proceedings of each have been published as a peer-reviewed or informal report. These documents have been widely distributed and are valued by environmental scientists, engineers, regulators, and managers because of their technical basis and their comprehensive, state-of-the-science reviews. The workshops in the Pellston Series are as follows:

- Estimating the Hazard of Chemical Substances to Aquatic Life. Pellston, Michigan, 13–17 June 1977. Proceedings published by the American Society for Testing and Materials, STP 657, in 1978.

- Analyzing the Hazard Evaluation Process. Waterville Valley, New Hampshire, 14–18 August 1978. Proceedings published by The American Fisheries Society in 1979.

- Biotransformation and Fate of Chemicals in the Aquatic Environment. Pellston, Michigan, 14–18 August 1979. Proceedings published by The American Society of Microbiology in 1980.

- Modeling the Fate of Chemicals in the Aquatic Environment. Pellston, Michigan, 16–21 August 1981. Proceedings published by Ann Arbor Science in 1982.

- Environmental Hazard Assessment of Effluents. Cody, Wyoming, 23–27 August 1982. Proceedings published in a SETAC Special Publication by Pergamon Press in 1986.

- Fate and Effects of Sediment-Bound in Aquatic Systems. Florissant, Colorado, 11–18 August 1984. Proceedings published in a SETAC Special Publication by Pergamon Press in 1987.

- Research Priorities in Environmental Risk Assessment. Breckenridge, Colorado, 16–21 August 1987. Proceedings published by SETAC in 1987.

- Biomarkers: Biochemical, Physiological, and Histological Markers of Anthropogenic Stress. Keystone, Colorado, 23–28 July 1989. Proceedings published in a SETAC Special Publication by Lewis Publishers in 1992.

- Population Ecology and Wildlife Toxicology of Agricultural Pesticide Use: A Modeling Initiative for Avian Species. Kiawah Island, South Carolina, 22–27 July 1990. Proceedings published in a SETAC Special Publication by Lewis Publishers in 1993.

- A Technical Framework for [Product] Life-Cycle Assessments. Smuggler's Notch, Vermont, 18–23 August 1990. Proceedings published by SETAC in January 1991, with second printing in September 1991 and third printing in March 1994.

- Aquatic Microcosms for Ecological Assessment of Pesticides. Wintergreen, Virginia, 7–11 October 1991. Final Report published February 1992.

- A Conceptual Framework for Life-Cycle Assessment Impact Assessment. Sandestin, Florida 1–6 February 1992. Proceedings published by SETAC in 1993.
- A Mechanistic Understanding of Bioavailability: Physical-Chemical Interactions. Pellston, Michigan, 17–22 August 1992. Proceedings published in a SETAC Special Publication by Lewis Publishers in 1994.
- Life-Cycle Assessment Data Quality Workshop. Wintergreen, Virginia, 4–9 October 1992. Proceedings published by SETAC in 1994.
- Avian Radio Telemetry in Support of Pesticide Field Studies. Pacific Grove, California, 5–8 January 1993. Proceedings to be published by SETAC in 1997.
- Sustainability-Based Environmental Management. Pellston, Michigan, 25–31 August 1993. Co-sponsored by the Ecological Society of America. Proceedings to be published by SETAC in 1997.
- Ecotoxicological Risk Assessment of Chlorinated Organic Chemicals. Alliston, Ontario, Canada, 25–29 July 1994. Proceedings to be published by SETAC in 1998.
- Application of Life-Cycle Assessment to Public Policy. Wintergreen, Virginia, 14–19 August 1994. Proceedings to be published by SETAC in 1997.
- Ecological Risk Assessment Modeling Systems. Pellston, Michigan, 23–28 August 1994. Proceedings to be published by SETAC in 1997.
- Avian Toxicity Testing. Pensacola, Florida, 4–7 December 1994. Co-sponsored by OECD. Proceedings published by OECD in 1996.
- Chemical Ranking and Scoring. Sandestin, Florida, 12–16 February 1995. Proceedings published by SETAC in 1997.
- Sediments Risk Assessment. Pacific Grove, California, 23–28 April 1995. Proceedings published by SETAC in 1997.
- Ecotoxicology and Risk Assessment for Wetlands. Gregson, Montana, 30 July–3 August 1995. Proceedings to be published by SETAC in 1998.
- Uncertainty in Ecological Risk Assessment. Pellston, Michigan, 23–28 August 1995. Proceedings to be published by SETAC in 1998.
- Whole-Effluent Toxicity. Pellston, Michigan, 16–21 September 1995. Proceedings published by SETAC in 1996.
- Reassessment of Metals Criteria for Aquatic Life Protection: Priorities for Research and Implementation. Pensacola, Florida, 10–14 February 1996. Proceedings published by SETAC in 1997.
- Reproductive and Developmental Effects in Oviparous Vertebrates. Gregson, Montana, 13–18 July 1977. Proceedings to be published by SETAC in 1998.

Information about the availability of workshop reports can be obtained by contacting

Society of Environmental Toxicology and Chemistry (SETAC)
1010 North 12th Avenue, Pensacola, FL 32501-3370 U.S.A.
T 850 469 1500   F 850 469 9778
E setac@setac.org   http://www.setac.org

SETAC Press

Preface

This book presents the proceedings of the 21st "Pellston Workshop," held 12–16 February 1995 at Sandestin, Florida. Like previous workshops, participation was limited to invited experts from government, academia, and industry who were selected because of their experience with the workshop topic. The workshop provided a structured environment for the exchange of ideas and debate such that consensus positions would be derived and documented for some of the issues surrounding the science of chemical ranking and scoring. The proceedings reflect the current state-of-the-art of these topics and focus on an assessment of 1) framework issues, 2) measures of exposure, 3) human health effects, 4) ecological effects, and 5) other chemical characteristics to consider in chemical ranking and scoring.

Acknowledgments

The Pellston Workshop on Chemical Ranking and Scoring and publication of the workshop proceedings were made possible through the financial support of the American Automobile Manufacturers Association, the Charles Stewart Mott Foundation, the Chemical Manufacturers Association, the Chlorine Chemicals Council, The Dow Chemical Company, Environment Canada, Health Canada, 3M Company, Monsanto Company, Rohm and Haas Company, E.I. du Pont deNemours and Company, and the U.S. Environmental Protection Agency (USEPA). The content of this publication does not necessarily reflect the position or the policy of any of these organizations or the United States government, and no official endorsement should be inferred.

The workshop organizers gratefully acknowledge the participants for their enthusiastic commitment to the workshop's objectives and for their cooperative efforts in the preparation of this book. We are also deeply indebted to the SETAC/SETAC Foundation Office staff and volunteers who contributed to the success of the workshop. Special thanks go to Greg Schiefer, Rod Parrish, Linda Longsworth, and Nancy Boykin for their hard work in planning and implementing the workshop and to Lisa Credeur for her diligence in preparing the final manuscript. We also greatly appreciate Chris Englert's and Mimi Meredith's valuable assistance in editing the manuscript throughout the review process. Special thanks also go to Margaret Goergen of the Center for Clean Products and Clean Technologies for assistance in preparing the many drafts of the manuscript.

Members of the CRS Workshop Steering Committee and Book Editing Committee are

- Gary A. Davis, University of Tennessee, Center for Clean Products and Clean Technologies: Steering Committee, Editing Committee
- James A. Fava, Roy F. Weston: Steering Committee
- Daniel Fort, USEPA, Office of Pollution Prevention and Toxics: Steering Committee, Editing Committee
- Emma Lou George, USEPA, Office of Research and Development: Steering Committee, Editing Committee
- Gary K. Hurlburt, Michigan Department of Natural Resources: Steering Committee, Editing Committee
- Frances H. Irwin, World Wildlife Fund: Steering Committee, Editing Committee
- Allan A. Jensen, dk-TEKNIK, Denmark: Steering Committee, Editing Committee
- Richard A. Kimerle, Monsanto Company: Steering Committee, Editing Committee
- Claudia O'Brien, USEPA, Office of Pollution Prevention and Toxics: Steering Committee
- Rodney Parrish, SETAC / SETAC Foundation: Steering Committee
- Gregory E. Schiefer, SETAC / SETAC Foundation: Steering Committee, Editing Committee

- Adam C. Socha, Ontario Ministry of the Environment and Energy: Editing Committee
- Mary B. Swanson, University of Tennessee, Center for Clean Products and Clean Technologies: Steering Committee, Editing Committee
- John D. Walker, USEPA, TSCA Interagency Testing Committee: Editing Committee

About the Editors

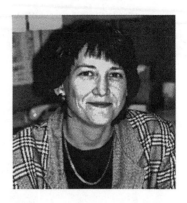

Mary B. Swanson is a Research Scientist with the University of Tennessee's Energy, Environment and Resources Center and the Center for Clean Products and Clean Technologies. Her work involves evaluating the fate and effects of chemicals released to the environment, with special interest in the development and application of chemical ranking and scoring, risk assessment, and life-cycle impact assessment methodologies as tools for evaluating and developing cleaner products and cleaner technologies.

Ms. Swanson has 12 years of experience in environmental research and consulting, beginning with research at the University of Minnesota involving trace organic contaminants in rain and snow in the Great Lakes region. Prior to UT, she worked in environmental consulting as an environmental chemist and environmental engineer on hazardous waste site remedial investigations and feasibility studies, specializing in contaminant fate and transport modeling and human health risk assessment.

Ms. Swanson received a Master of Science degree in environmental engineering from the University of Minnesota in 1988 and a Bachelor of Science degree in natural resources/water chemistry from the University of Wisconsin-Stevens Point in 1984.

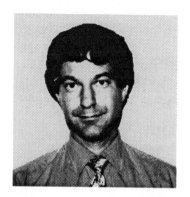

Adam C. Socha's present position is Senior Advisor, Regulatory Toxicology in the Environmental Standards Section, Standards Development Branch, Ontario Ministry of Environment and Energy (OMOEE), Toronto, Ontario, Canada.

Mr. Socha has served as a toxicologist and technical manager with the OMOEE for over 10 years. Part of his work has involved the development and application of hazard scoring, screening, and ranking methods for the OMOEE and for Canada's government/industry "ARET" voluntary toxic substance elimination and reduction program. He has also been a consultant in the development and application of scoring and ranking systems by Environment Canada, Health Canada, the Michigan Department of Environmental Quality, and the U.S./Canada Great Lakes Binational Objectives Development Committee. During 1995, Mr. Socha had an external secondment to CAW Canada (Canadian Auto Workers Union), where he developed environmental policy and provided advice and training to union members on environmental and occupational health matters.

Mr. Socha received his Bachelor of Science degree in pharmacology and toxicology from the University of Toronto in 1983 and his Master of Science degree in toxicology and physiology from the Ontario Veterinary College, University of Guelph, in 1986.

Workshop Participants and Contributing Authors

(by work group and chapter editor)

Framework Issues

Gary Davis (chapter editor), Dan Fort, Bjørn Hansen, Fran Irwin, Baxter Jones, Sheila Jones, Adam Socha, Robert Wilson, Bill Haaf, George Gray, Bill Hoffman

Measures of Exposure

Mary Swanson (chapter editor), Bob Boethling, John Evans, John Geisy, Jim Gillett, Phil Howard, David Jeffrey, Jay Jon, Preben Kristensen, Robert Larson, Yong-Hwa Kim

Human Health Effects

Gary Hurlburt (chapter editor), Rolf Bretz, Emma Lou George, Rolf Hartung, Ray Kent, Lynne Fahey McGrath, Ron Newhook, Mike Stevens, Brad Strohm, Pauline Wagner

Ecological Effects

Rich Kimerle (chapter editor), Larry Barnthouse, Richard Brown, Bernard Conilh de Beyssac, Mike Gilbertson, Kathy Monk, Heinz-Jochen Poremski, Richard Purdy, Kevin Reinert, Rosalind Rolland, Maurice Zeeman

Other Chemical Characteristics

Allan A. Jensen and John Walker (chapter editors), Franz Fiala, Karim Ahmed, Mark Ralston, Robert Ross, Friedrich Schmidt-Bleek, Duane Tolle

SETAC Press

Introduction

With increasingly limited resources in business and government, one of the most important problems facing decision-makers is the allocation and prioritization of resources. There is a need for tools that can provide information on the human health and environmental hazards posed by chemical releases from industrial facilities, products, or hazardous material sites. There is also a growing recognition of the need for consistent decisions across governmental programs as well as increased attention to selection of materials based on environmental attributes in the contexts of product stewardship, life-cycle assessment, and pollution prevention.

Given these needs, it is not surprising that there is a large and growing number of people interested in and using chemical ranking and scoring (CRS), with a diversity of goals, across a broad spectrum of industry, government, and academia. Uses of CRS include regulatory action, evaluating the potential impacts of chemical releases, and priority setting 1) on testing or additional analysis, 2) among risk reduction opportunities, and 3) for pollution prevention activities.

There is also a need for agreement and valid CRS methods. Hundreds of CRS systems have been developed in the past 20 years. The structures of these ranking and scoring systems vary widely, with no consensus on the scientific and technical framework underpinning those methods. Consensus is needed for consistency across regulatory programs in air, water, waste site, and product approvals and among various regulatory agencies at state, national, and international levels.

During the last decade, methods used to assess chemical toxicity and environmental fate have made vast improvements. Chemical ranking and scoring combines an assessment of both the toxic effects of chemicals (human and/or environmental) and the potential exposure to those chemicals to provide a relative evaluation of risk. Often, ranking and scoring systems are part of an iterative approach to risk assessment and risk management.

There is also little available guidance for developing or using CRS tools. Ideally, a CRS system would be chosen based upon the goals of the evaluation for which it is used, the level of information desired, the degree of acceptable uncertainty, and the available resources with a clear system output that relates to the desired goal. Users need to choose those systems that yield output that meets their needs rather than to tailor their needs to a system's output.

The objectives of the CRS workshop were
- to bring together people who are currently working in the area of CRS;
- to characterize the current state of the science;
- based on the principles of human health and ecological risk assessment, to develop a consensus on the scientific and technical framework for CRS to

promote consistency in the development and application of CRS systems among government, industry, academia, and environmental groups;

- to develop guidelines and principles for CRS; and
- to define research necessary to fill data and methodological gaps.

With these aims, a SETAC-sponsored workshop on CRS was held 12–16 February 1995, in Sandestin, Florida. Fifty-one experts were brought together from the United States, Austria, Canada, Denmark, Germany, Italy, the United Kingdom, Switzerland, and South Korea. Participants were from government, industry, academic institutions, and nongovernmental and environmental organizations. Five working groups evaluated framework issues, methods for assessing exposure, human health effects, ecological effects, and other chemical characteristics within the context of CRS.

This document presents the current status of CRS and the workshop consensus on the framework for CRS for effects and exposure. It includes recommended principles developed as guidance for those applying an existing CRS system or developing a new CRS system to meet specific goals.

The workshop steering committee saw a framework for CRS as a first step in a program to develop a broad consensus for overall human health and environmental risk ranking. Hopefully, a program on CRS will follow that will ultimately build consensus on some of the more detailed scientific issues and guide the development of a consensus CRS system or systems.

Executive Summary

Chemical ranking and scoring (CRS) is a tool for assessing chemicals by considering health effects, environmental effects or other hazards, persistence, and exposure. Chemical ranking and scoring either produces a relative ranking of chemicals or assigns chemicals to specific groups or categories. Hundreds of CRS systems have been developed in the past 20 years. Industry, governmental agencies, and academia have developed CRS systems for direct regulatory or risk management action, priority setting for further investigation, and impact evaluation. To date, there has been little guidance for developing these systems, and methods vary widely.

The Society of Environmental Toxicology and Chemistry (SETAC) sponsored a Chemical Ranking and Scoring Workshop, held 12–16 February 1995, in Sandestin, Florida. Fifty-one experts were brought together from Austria, Canada, Denmark, Germany, Italy, the United Kingdom, Switzerland, South Korea, and the United States. Participants represented government agencies, industry, academic institutions, and nongovernmental and environmental organizations. The goal of the workshop was to develop a consensus framework, along with principles, to promote consistency in the development and application of CRS systems.

Workshop Results

Five working groups addressed framework issues and technical elements of methods for assessing exposure potential, human health effects, ecological effects, and other chemical characteristics. Results of the plenary and workgroup sessions include 1) documenting current and emerging uses of CRS and the state of the science, 2) identifying key issues in CRS, and 3) developing principles to serve as guidance for those applying an existing CRS system or developing a new CRS system for a specific purpose.

The general findings of the workshop are that CRS systems
- are not quantitative risk assessments but, if constructed properly, are part of the risk assessment paradigm;
- are important tools in risk management;
- do not exist in a single form that fits all uses and applications;
- need not proliferate unless a unique application requires a new or revised approach; and
- can be particularly useful tools where resources are limited for chemical risk assessment and risk management.

Current and Emerging Uses of CRS

There are many current and potential CRS applications. One important application is for regulatory and risk management purposes. For example, regulators use CRS to develop lists of chemicals for reporting and monitoring those chemicals that may threaten state or regional water quality and to select chemicals for bans or phaseout. Other applications include priority setting for testing, assessment, and determining pollution prevention priorities. Industry uses CRS to set priorities for research and development, to focus product stewardship activities, and to determine chemical data needs.

Chemical ranking and scoring is potentially a very useful tool in the impact assessment stage of life-cycle assessment (LCA), to evaluate how inventoried releases might impact human health and the environment. Chemical ranking and scoring is also emerging as a tool for waste minimization activities. For example, high priority waste streams can be evaluated to determine the technical and economic feasibility of source reduction and recycling alternatives. Governments of many developing countries are facing increased demands to provide environmental protection; CRS can assist regulators and risk managers to expand existing environmental quality standards and to develop new standards.

The General Framework

Given the wide variety of uses, there is no single CRS system appropriate to all applications. The primary goal of the workshop was to develop agreement on the basic scientific framework of CRS systems. It was hoped that this would promote consistency among current and future CRS systems. One of the goals of a CRS framework is to promote consistency and harmonization so that the various CRS methods used are universally recognizable and employ similar principles. Workshop participants developed guiding principles to improve development and application of CRS. They also identified broad goals of any CRS system:

- **Organize and transmit information** by transforming chemical data into a form that can be presented clearly and consistently to the intended audience. In doing so, a CRS system will facilitate communication among industry, government, academia, environmental advocacy groups, and the public.

- **Provide information for management activities** using the available information to differentiate chemicals from each other and to show their relative human health, ecological, or other impacts. Chemical ranking and scoring should be used to protect human health and the environment, guide the development of safer products, promote safer substitutes, and improve the safety of materials in products. A CRS system should communicate uncertainty and increase understanding of the confidence level of the ranking or scoring, thereby increasing the confidence in decisions about chemicals.

Principles of CRS system development

The following principles apply to the development of any new CRS system and to the selection of an existing system for a particular application. In developing these principles, the workshop participants recognized that CRS used for different applications may have different forms and degrees of complexity. Regardless of the application, however, a CRS system should

- have a clearly defined purpose;
- include both effects and exposure data, as is consistent with the risk assessment paradigm;
- acknowledge and assess uncertainty;
- acknowledge the role of professional judgment;
- consider effects relevant to the goals;
- recognize the role of valuation in aggregation and weighting of different endpoints;
- have transparent methods and outputs;
- be neutral to data availability, unless it is consistent with the intended use to have a positive or negative bias;
- accommodate extreme data variability across chemicals;
- use a tiered approach;
- assess similar effects/exposure categories consistently across tiers;
- preserve critical information;
- specify data selection guidelines;
- be theory-driven as well as data-driven;
- include sensitivity analysis;
- be consistent with any pre-selection of chemicals; and
- consider the impacts of scaling.

A generic CRS framework

The generic framework for CRS consists of 4 primary steps:

1) **Goal definition and scoping:** The goals of a CRS system are determined by the risk management goals of the process (i.e., what decisions will be made based on the CRS results) and should be defined at the outset. Scoping involves identifying the starting point, methods used to process the information, and any tiers that might be used.
2) **Indicator selection:** This involves the identification of the type and amount of data needed for the particular CRS exercise.
3) **Ranking and scoring:** This should be based on agreed-upon principles.
4) **Output and presentation:** The results should be reported in a form useful for achieving the goal of the analysis.

Technical Working Groups

Four of the five working groups evaluated the technical aspects of exposure, human health effects, ecological effects, and other chemical characteristics in CRS. This section summarizes the results of these working groups' efforts.

Exposure assessment methods

There are many different CRS methods to assess exposure. These methods vary in 2 basic ways. First, they are either generic or site-specific. Second, the exposure measures used vary from simple surrogate measures to more sophisticated estimates of environmental concentrations or human-dose rates. Workgroup recommendations include the following:

- The scope (i.e., number of factors pertaining to exposure that are considered) and analytical sophistication of the exposure assessment in a CRS system should be determined based on the acceptable degree of uncertainty for the decisions that are to be made.
- A sequential (or tiered) approach should be used, applying the simplest methods first. For instance, a preliminary score might be developed based on a highly aggregated analysis involving only 2 or 3 parameters; more sophisticated second- or third-tier estimates would be applied only if determined necessary by a previous screening step. The structure should contain feedback loops to trigger further analysis of potentially important chemicals.
- Environmental fate parameters should include molecular weight, water solubility, octanol- water partition coefficient (Kow) or organic carbon partition coefficient (Koc), vapor pressure, Henry's Law constant, acid dissociation constant (pKa), aquatic bioconcentration factor (BCF), and chemical persistence.

Human health effects

A fundamental problem for any CRS system is summarizing the large number of human health effects that are investigated in laboratory, clinical, and epidemiological studies. Three broad types of effects should be considered in CRS: acute toxicity, subchronic/chronic toxicity, and carcinogenicity. The specific intended use of the system will determine which of these effects should be included.

Modifying factors should be used to adjust measures of hazard that are not adequately represented by the 3 effect endpoints alone. These are qualitative factors related to hazard, and their application requires professional judgment. These modifiers include

- the severity of the effect,
- how extensively the chemical has been tested,
- the quality of the data used to derive scores in each of the 3 effect categories,
- chemical potency for the effect being considered, and
- mutagenic/genotoxic potential.

Ecological effects

The assessment of ecological effects is an essential component of CRS. Aquatic and terrestrial environments are the primary areas of concern. Organisms of ecological interest that generally have available toxicity data include algae, invertebrates, fish, birds, and domestic or laboratory mammals. Also of ecological interest are effects data on species that offer some understanding of potential impacts on terrestrial wildlife mammals, birds, reptiles, and amphibians. The endpoint of primary interest is the no-observable-effects concentration (NOEC). Measured data are preferred, but the NOEC can also be derived from the more readily available acute data. Data obtained from quantitative structure-activity relationship (QSAR) studies are generally useful, obtainable, and important as a source of data for chemical screening.

There is no definitive "right" scoring procedure for ecological effects. Rather, there are alternative approaches depending on the purpose of scoring. Procedures addressed by the working group include
1) prescreening with much scientific judgment;
2) screening of threshold effects data with no consideration of exposure (hazard ranking);
3) use of ordinal assignments of data (scores) compiled in an algorithm that weights components; and
4) application of a risk-based quotient approach using exposure, effects, and a margin of safety.

A useful initial screening approach includes the broad ecological effects parameters of persistence, bioaccumulation, and aquatic toxicity.

Other chemical characteristics

Chemical releases may result in impacts not typically accounted for in CRS systems. Other important characteristics include the following:
- chemical properties (e.g., flammability, corrosivity);
- chemical–environmental interactions (e.g., ozone depletion, odor, global warming);
- waste reduction and management (e.g., source reduction, ability to detect chemicals in waste); and
- material resources, energy use, and land use associated with chemical production.

The extent to which these characteristics are incorporated into a CRS system depends on the scope of the CRS process. Methods for quantifying these other characteristics require further development if they are to be used in CRS systems. Some areas are more developed and already are used in CRS systems (e.g., physical effects and global/regional impacts), while other areas require further work or research (e.g., waste management and resource productivity).

Research Needs and Recommendations for Future Work

Many research needs concern data availability and how new data can be incorporated as they become available. General recommendations are as follows:

- Develop a common, readily available database that includes physical-chemical properties, intrinsic exposure-related data, and toxicological data. This would greatly reduce the amount of time required to conduct CRS and would improve consistency among applications.
- Develop methods to address the effects of chemical mixtures of substances on human health and the environment.
- Improve communication and coordination among CRS practitioners in international organizations and the U.S., including state and federal agencies.
- Maintain, in a central location, an inventory of CRS systems currently in use and those developed in the future, to ensure current and accessible information for CRS practitioners.
- Categorize and recommend CRS methods for prioritizing chemicals for testing, designing safer substitutes, and assessing risks to workers, consumers or general populations.
- Recommend CRS methods that can be cost-effectively employed by developing countries.

Other areas of CRS in need of further work or research include the following:

- For exposure, develop methods to treat uncertainty and variability, and determine methods appropriate to different applications and differing data quality needs (levels of acceptable uncertainty).
- For human health effects, develop methods to use epidemiologic data, incorporate new test methods as they become available (e.g., in vitro skin and eye irritation studies), and consider metabolism as well as the mode of action of chemical toxicity.
- For ecological effects, consider the mode of action by which chemicals elicit effects, the effects of chemical exposure via soil, and the effects of chemicals on higher aquatic and terrestrial plants, photoinduced toxicity, and neurotoxicity.
- For other chemical characteristics, further develop criteria for evaluating physical/chemical properties (e.g., flammability/ignitability, explosivity/reactivity, oxidation, and corrosivity); develop methods to quantify and include alteration-of-environment effects (e.g., global warming, ozone depletion, photochemical oxidation, odor, eutrophication, and acidification); improve/develop methods for ranking resource productivity; and evaluate the impact of including other effects in a CRS system.

Future Activities

Suggestions for future CRS activities include the following:

- Establish a SETAC advisory-type committee for CRS.
- Hold follow-up CRS workshops to further the work of this first CRS workshop. Suggested subjects include aggregation and weighting issues and assessing human and ecological exposure.
- Establish and maintain a database or other compilation of CRS methods and applications.
- Hold an open forum in Washington DC to present conclusions and recommendations from this workshop.

Abbreviations

ACGIH	American Conference of Governmental Industrial Hygienists
AP	acidification potential
AQUIRE	Aquatic Toxicity Information Retrieval database
ARET	Accelerated Reduction/Elimination of Toxics
ASFA	Aquatic Science and Fisheries Abstracts
ASTER	Assessment Tools for the Evaluation of Risk
ATSDR	Agency for Toxic Substances and Disease Registry
BAF	bioaccumulation factor
BCF	bioconcentration factor
BOD	biological oxygen demand
BP	boiling point
BRS	biennial reporting system
BUA	Beratergremium für Umweltrelevante Altstoffe
CANCERLIT	Cancer Literature database
CAS	Chemical Abstracts Service
CASE	computer automated structure evaluation
CA SEARCH	Chemical Abstracts Search
CCINFO	Canadian Centre for Occupational Health and Safety Information system
CCRIS	Chemical Carcinogenesis Research Information System
CERCLA	Comprehensive Environmental Response, Compensation & Liability Act
CESARS	Chemical Evaluation Search and Retrieval System
CCOHS	Canadian Centre for Occupational Health & Safety
CHEMFATE	Chemical Fate database
CHEMINFO	Chemical Information database
CHEMS-1	Chemical Hazard Evaluation for Management Strategies
CIS	Chemical Information System
CMR	Critical Materials Register
COD	chemical oxygen demand
CRGS	Chemical Regulations and Guidelines System
CRS	chemical ranking and scoring
DART	Developmental and Reproductive Toxicity database
DDT	dichlorodiphenyl trichloroethane
DF	degradation factor

DHL	degradation half-life
DO	dissolved oxygen
DOC	dissolved organic carbon
DWEL	drinking water exposure limit
EC	European Commission
EC50	effective concentration to 50% of a test population
ECB	European Chemicals Bureau
ECOSAR	Ecotoxicity of Industrial Chemicals Based on Structure-Activity Relationships
ECOTOX	Ecotoxicology database
ED10	effective dose causing a response in 10% of a test population
EEC	European Economic Community
EEDB	Environmental Effects DataBase
EFDB	Environmental Fate DataBase
ELHILL	E.L. Hill Computer System, U.S. National Library of Medicine
EMBASE	Excerpta Medica database
EMPPL	Effluent Monitoring Priority Pollutants List (Ontario)
ENVIROFATE	Environmental Fate database
EP	eutrophication potential
EPI©	Estimation Programs Interface
EPS	Environmental Priority Strategies
EU	European Union
fa	fraction of chemical in air
fb	fraction of chemical in biotic compartment
fso	fraction of chemical in soil
fs	fraction of chemical in sediment
fw	fraction of chemical in water
FEL	frank effect levels
FP	flash point
GENETOX	Genotoxicity database
GLP	good laboratory practice
GWU	George Washington University
GWP	global warming potential
Hc	Henry's Law constant
HC	hydrocarbon
HEAST	Health Effects Assessment Summary Tables
HEDSET	Harmonized Electronic DataSet

HRS	hazard ranking system
HSDB	Hazardous Substances Data Bank
IARC	International Agency for Research on Cancer
IC50	inhibitory concentration to 50% of exposed population
IPCC	International Panel on Climate Change
IPPW	Identifiers, Production, Processes, and Waste (IRPTC)
IPS	Informal Working Group on Priority Setting
IRIS	Integrated Risk Information System
IRPTC	International Registry of Potentially Toxic Chemicals
ISHOW	Information System for Hazardous Organics in Water
ITC	Interagency Testing Committee
IUCLID	International Uniform Chemical Information Database
IUPAC	International Union of Physicists and Chemists
k_1	first order degradation rate constant
kb	first order degradation rate
Kd	chemical soil–water partitioning coefficient
Koc	organic carbon–water partition coefficient
Kow	octanol–water partition coefficient
L	liter
LC50	lethal concentration to 50% of test population
LC_{LO}	lowest lethal concentration
LCA	life-cycle assessment
LD1	lethal dose to 1% of test population
LD10	lethal dose to 10% of test population
LD50	lethal dose to 50% of test population
LD_{LO}	lowest lethal dose
LFER	linear free energy relationship
LOAEC	lowest-observed-adverse-effect concentration
LOAEL	lowest-observed-adverse-effect level
MATC	maximum allowable toxicant concentration
MCA	multi-criteria analysis
MCMR	Michigan Critical Materials Register
MCNR	Michigan Department of Natural Resources
MED	Mid-Continent Ecology Division (USEPA)
MEDLARS	Medical Literature Access and Retrieval System (U.S. National Library of Medicine)
MEDLINE	Medical Information On-Line (U.S. National Library of Medicine)

μeq	microequivalents
μg	microgram
mg	milligrams
MI	material intensity
MIPS	material intensity per unit service
MISA	municipal–industrial strategy for abatement
MIXTOX	Mixture Toxicity Estimation System (USEPA)
MLD	minimum lethal dose
MLE	maximum likelihood estimate
MPD	minimum Premarket Data Set
MSDS	Material Safety Data Sheet
MUSEPAS	Multimedia Environmental Pollutant Assessment System
MW	molecular weight
NAS	National Academy of Science
NFPA	National Fire Prevention Association
NHATS	National Human Adipose Tissue Survey
NIOSH	National Institute for Occupational Safety and Health
NOAA	National Oceanic and Atmospheric Administration
NOAEC	no-observed-adverse-effect concentration
NOAEL	no-observed-adverse-effect level
NOEC	no-observed-effect concentration
NOEL	no-observed effect level
NOES	National Occupational Exposure Survey
NPDES	National Pollutant Discharge Elimination System
NPIRS	National Pesticide Information Retrieval System
NPL	National Priority List
NTIS	National Technical Information System
ODP	ozone depletion potential
OECD	Organization for Economic Cooperation and Development
OHM/TADS	Oil and Hazardous Materials/Technical Assistance Data System
OMOEE	Ontario Ministry of Environment and Energy (formerly Ontario Ministry of Environment [OMOE])
OPPT	USEPA Office of Pollution Prevention and Toxics (formerly OTS)
OSHA	U.S. Occupational Safety and Health Administration
OSW	Office of Solid Waste (USEPA)
OTS	Office of Toxic Substances
OTV	odor threshold values

PAN	peroxyl acetyl nitrate
PBT	persistent, bioaccumulative, and toxic
PCB	polychlorinated biphenyl
PEL	permissible exposure limit
PETN	pentaerythritol tetranitrate
PHYSPROP	Physical Properties database
PHYTOTOX	Phytotoxicology database
pKa	dissociation constant
PNEC	predicted no-effect concentration
POCP	photochemical oxidant creation potential
ppm	parts per million
PRIS	Pesticide Research Information System (Information Canada)
PTRRs	pollutant transfer and release registries
PUD	production, use, and disposal
Pv	vapor pressure
QRA	quantitative risk assessment
QSAR	quantitative structure-activity relationship
RAPS	Remedial Action Priority System
RCRA	U.S. Resource Conservation and Recovery Act
RD50	concentration that elicits a 50% reduction in respiratory rate
RfC	reference concentration
RfD	reference dose
RI	risk index
RIPP	Regulatory Information on Pesticide Products (Canada)
RIVM	National Institute of Public Health and Environmental Protection (Netherlands)
RPA	resource productivity analysis
RQ	reportable quantity (Chapters 1, 3, 5); risk quotient (Chapter 4)
RREL	Risk Reduction Engineering Laboratory (USEPA)
RT	residence time
RTECS	Registry of Toxic Effects of Chemical Substances (NIOSH)
s	mean score
S	water solubility
SANSS	Structure and Nomenclature Search System
SAR	structure-activity relationship
SARA	Superfund Amendments and Reauthorization Act
SAT	Structure-activity Team
SCISEARCH	Science Information Search System

SETAC	Society of Environmental Toxicology and Chemistry
SIC	standard industrial classification
SIDS	Screening Information Data Set
SMILES	Simplified Molecular Line Input System
SRC	Syracuse Research Corporation
STN	Science and Technical Network
SuCCSES	Substructure-based Computerized Chemical Selection Expert System
T	time
$t_{1/2}$	environmental half-life
TERRETOX	Terrestrial Toxicology database
THOD	theoretical oxygen demand
TLV	threshold limit value
TOXLINE	Toxicology Information On-Line
TOXNET	Toxicology Data Network
TRI	Toxics Release Inventory
TRIGRAS	Toxics Release Inventory Geographic Risk Analysis System
TSCA	U.S. Toxic Substances Control Act
TSCAPP	Toxic Substances Control Act Plant and Production Search System
TSCATS	Toxic Substances Control Act Test Submissions database
U.S.	United States
UCSS	Use Cluster Scoring System
USBLS	U.S. Bureau of Labor Statistics
USEPA	U.S. Environmental Protection Agency
USES	Uniform System for the Evaluation of Substances
USHEW	U.S. Department of Health Education and Welfare
UT	University of Tennessee
UV	ultraviolet
UV-B	biologically harmful ultraviolet
VOC	volatile organic compound
WMPT	Waste Minimization Prioritization Tool
WMS	Wet Milieugevaarlijke Stoffen (substances dangerous to the environment)
WOE	weight of evidence

Chapter 1

Framework for Chemical Ranking and Scoring Systems

Gary Davis, chapter editor
Dan Fort, Bjørn Hansen, Fran Irwin, Baxter Jones, Sheila Jones,
Adam Socha, Robert Wilson, Bill Haaf, George Gray, Bill Hoffman

Chemical ranking and scoring (CRS) is a tool to provide practical information on human health and environmental hazards, exposure, and/or risk of chemicals for risk management decisions. A key advantage of CRS systems is that they can conserve resources by tailoring the analysis to the decision at hand. For example, CRS can be used for identifying and prioritizing chemicals for further study or risk assessment, comparing alternative chemicals for industrial processes for resource allocation, or setting priorities among risk reduction opportunities.

Goals of a Chemical Ranking and Scoring Framework

The overall goal of the Pellston Workshop on Chemical Ranking and Scoring was to develop a consensus CRS framework. There are 3 primary goals for a CRS framework:

1) to promote consistency and harmonization among CRS methods,

2) to provide a structure for organizing and transmitting information, and

3) to improve the means of providing information for management activities.

Promote consistency and harmonization

Clearly one of the goals of a broad CRS framework is to start the process of harmonizing the large number of scoring systems currently in use. This does not mean that all systems should use the same scoring methodology but rather that the various methods used should be universally recognizable and should employ similar principles.

Organize and transmit information

A CRS system should be able to organize and translate the often confusing wealth of data on a bewildering number of chemicals into a form that can be presented clearly and consistently to the intended audience. In doing so, a CRS system will facilitate communication about chemicals among industry, government, academia, and the public. There are several elements to the goal of transmitting information: the audience, the goals of the study, and the form of the presentation.

One paradox of CRS is that a complete set of information about one particular chemical may be difficult to find, yet there is some limited information available for many thousands of chemicals. Before discussion about the issues of chemical use, regulation, or further testing can begin, these data must be summarized or otherwise condensed into an understandable and useful format. This may take the form of tables, graphs, groupings, or other visual aids. It also requires the content to be relevant to the discussion.

The information produced should be able to support the purpose of the study, whether the goal is risk management, community outreach, life-cycle impact assessment, or priority setting for further testing and data collection. Defining the goal and purpose of the study before beginning the collection of data should save time and help to ensure that the results produced by the system are commensurate with the goal and purpose. For example, if a particular CRS system is used to assess the human and ecological impacts of toxic chemical releases for a life-cycle assessment (LCA), the results will need to be in the same units as the rest of the impact assessment, whether the units are expressed as environmental points, dollars, or risk.

Provide information for management activities

In general, a CRS system provides information about the relative or comparative exposure, hazard, or risk posed by chemicals to assist in allocation of resources in a resource-constrained world. This information can aid in risk management decisions or in setting priorities for further assessment, testing, or data collection.

If the CRS system does not adequately differentiate between the chemicals being scored or ranked, it will be impossible to use the system to make management decisions. For instance, a system that ranks chemicals separately by human health effects and ecological effects but provides no method to compare or combine the results may not provide adequate information for risk management. At the same time, a system that lacks refinement and categorizes most of the chemicals scored in the same class gives the user little useful information.

Use of CRS can help guide the development of cleaner products and improve the management of chemicals used in manufacturing. Governments, or manufacturers themselves, can develop lists of restricted materials or preferred materials that can guide the choice of materials for product manufacturing. Materials can be clustered by use and compared to each other to determine the material for a particular use that poses the least overall risk. Cleaner product design can also be aided by using chemical scoring information to estimate the overall hazard or risk associated with the materials in a finished product.

A CRS should make apparent the confidence level of the ranking that it generates to inform the user about the appropriate level of confidence in the subsequent decisions made about the ranked chemicals. Uncertainty associated with the ranking of chemicals is not addressed in most of the systems currently in use. This reflects in part the difficulty of determining uncertainty. Determining and communicating uncertainty is, however, an important element of the CRS framework.

The Chemical Ranking and Scoring Conceptual Framework

The conceptual framework for CRS describes how CRS fits within the larger field of chemical risk assessment and risk management. It also describes a generic framework applicable to any CRS system.

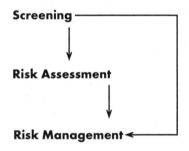

Figure 1-1   Chemical ranking/scoring and risk management

Ranking and scoring systems may provide information for risk management directly or indirectly, depending on the use and scope of the analysis (Figure 1-1). It is possible that either a CRS system leads directly to a risk management action or a CRS system identifies substances for further data collection and/or risk assessment. The critical factor is that CRS is conducted in order to provide relevant, useful information for risk management or other decision-making.

The risk assessment paradigm

Chemical ranking and scoring is consistent with, but not identical to, the concept of risk assessment. It is recognized that the potential threat posed by a chemical is a function of both hazard and exposure (National Academy of Sciences [NAS] 1983; USEPA 1984a). Therefore, although it may be appropriate to use only exposure or hazard information for some uses of CRS, most decisions will likely require an integration of both potential exposure and hazard information.

Chemical ranking and scoring is not generally considered equivalent to chemical risk assessment, although given the wide variety of CRS systems and approaches, no clear distinction between CRS and risk assessment can be made. Rather, the information needs and complexity of different CRS applications may be thought of as a continuum from simple, single-factor screening to quantitative risk assessment (QRA). Chemical ranking and scoring can employ QRA methodologies (e.g., when the evaluation includes site-specific exposure assessment and endpoint-specific assessment of potential effects based upon the hazard and exposure assessments). Most often, a few endpoints representing human health and environmental effects are evaluated, along with a relatively simple representation of potential for exposure. For instance, acute mammalian toxicity combined with carcinogenicity (to represent human health effects) and physical–chemical properties such as the octanol–water partition coefficient (to represent persistence in the environment) can be used as a simple chemical screening tier.

Chemical ranking and scoring is often performed in tiers with increasingly sophisticated levels of analysis and increased data needs moving from one tier to the next. The tiered approach (Figure 1-2) is often used to screen chemicals from one tier to the next to reduce the number of chemicals for which the increasingly sophisticated analysis and increased supporting data are necessary. The example in the preceding paragraph represents one of the first tiers. An example of a tier that requires more sophisticated analysis

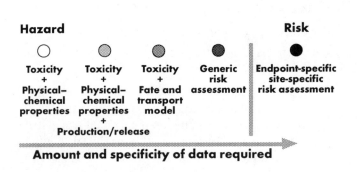

Figure 1-2 Chemical ranking and scoring conceptual framework

and more data would be one that combined several human health and environmental impact endpoints with a fate and transport analysis for each chemical to obtain a more detailed picture of potential effects.

A generic framework for chemical ranking and scoring

A generic framework for CRS (Figure 1-3) consists of 4 primary steps:

1) goal definition and scoping,

2) indicator selection,

3) ranking and scoring, and

4) output and presentation.

Goal definition and scoping are critical steps in CRS. Goal definition is determined by the risk management objective of the CRS process and will depend, in part, on the consequences of the decision. Identifying chemicals to study further would likely require a different scope and confidence level than identifying candidates for a government-imposed ban. Goal definition leads to scoping, which may be thought of as identifying the position on the CRS continuum for the analysis. This includes the starting point and any tiers that might be used. In addition, the methods that will be used to process the information are defined in this step. This goal definition and scoping step drives the rest of the CRS process, determining what data are needed, how they are organized and used, and how they are presented.

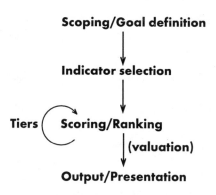

Figure 1-3 *Generic framework for chemical ranking and scoring*

Indicator selection involves identifying the type and amount of data needed for the particular CRS. The types of toxicological and exposure information will be influenced by the position on the continuum identified in the scoping step. The purpose of indicator selection is to use the appropriate types and levels of data to adequately inform risk managers and other decision-makers.

The ranking and scoring step is where the analysis actually occurs. The method by which the data are used to score and/or rank chemicals is defined as part of the scoping and goal definition stage. The process may be simple, such as placing chemicals in categories based on a few endpoints, or more complicated, involving numeric scoring and ranking methods.

The ranking and scoring step may be tiered. The use of tiers is a way to refine the analysis to increase efficiency and conserve resources. Common types of tiers reduce the number of chemicals that are addressed as the complexity of data and of the analysis applied to the chemicals is increased. Using tiers is essentially moving closer on the continuum to QRA with successive steps of analysis. The type and number of tiers depends on the scope and goals of the CRS process.

"Output/Presentation" in Figure 1-3 refers to the way in which the results of the CRS are put into a useful form. It is important to remember that the users of a CRS system may differ from the analysts. This means that an effort must be made to make the process transparent and to communicate important information to the user. Output of the CRS should include both the results of the process and a description of important assumptions and factors. This means that the risk manager will receive more information than simply a chemical's rank or score. There must also be a description of the methods used in the analysis. This should include factors considered and omitted, screens and tiers used, and important assumptions (e.g., how data gaps were treated). Additional quantitative information should include an aggregation of results as appropriate for the goals of the analysis, sensitivity analysis, and most importantly, a description of uncertainty in the analysis (major sources and potential influences). Any efforts to validate the results should also be discussed.

Types and Uses of Chemical Ranking and Scoring Systems

Types of chemical ranking and scoring systems

Many different types of chemical ranking systems have been developed and used. The most common types of systems can be classified broadly as

- simple categorizations based on expert judgment;
- decision rule with predefined criteria;
- endpoint scoring, with or without numerical aggregation; and
- generic risk calculation.

Within each class, there are numerous variants of system structure, and many existing systems are actually hybrids of these broad classes. Table 1-1 shows a classification of chemical ranking systems into 7 types (within the above 4 classes), briefly describes each type, and provides examples of systems fitting into each type.

All of these basic system types have potential applications in chemical ranking, and a single type of system cannot be demonstrated to be clearly superior for all uses. Each has certain advantages and disadvantages, and the system developer/user should consider these before developing or using a particular system. For example, endpoint scoring and generic risk calculation systems are typically (but not always) more complex and data- and resource-intensive than decision rule or simple categorization systems. This is because they often include more endpoints and integrate them to a greater degree. They also usually require more time and/or resources to develop and use, and consensus on the results may be difficult to achieve. In addition, complex endpoint scoring systems with many scoring elements tend to be less transparent than decision rule or simple categorization systems. Decision rule approaches allow sorting chemicals into groups based on multiple criteria without numerical aggregation of diverse endpoints. This aids in the transparency of these systems.

Simple categorization approaches incorporating expert judgment can frequently be developed and applied relatively quickly, which can be a significant advantage in some applications, but these approaches often suffer from lack of widespread acceptance of the results by parties external to the process. Thus, they are most useful for initial tiers of multitiered processes in which initial ranking decisions are confirmed in subsequent tiers.

Systems employing QRA methods have a limited range of application in CRS primarily because of their complexity and the issues related to reducing the exposure assessment component to a necessary level of simplicity. A key advantage of these systems, however, is that they most closely correspond to the general risk assessment paradigm that is being approximated by chemical ranking systems.

Table 1-1 Types of chemical ranking systems

Type of system	Description	Examples
Expert judgment/ categorization	Sorting chemicals into groups purely by expert opinion; can be one or multiple experts.	1) United States Environmental Protection Agency (USEPA) structure-activity team determinations
Checkoff/ categorization	Sorting chemicals into groups based on simple yes/no checkoff of pre-defined toxicity criteria and professional judgment.	1) DuPont internal system (Haaf 1995)
Decision rule	Sorting chemicals into groups based on pre-defined criteria (quantitative or qualitative), with pre-defined decision rules. Decision rules can be based on one criterion, multiple criteria in sequence, or multiple criteria in combination (e.g., "High" if a carcinogen **or** if LD50<1 mg/kg **and** releases >100,000 pounds).	1) Michigan Critical Materials Register (MCMR) approach (MDNR 1987) 2) Great Lakes Sunsetting (Foran and Glenn 1993) 3) Various chemical listing systems
Endpoint scoring, without numerical aggregation	Numerical scoring of each endpoint assessed, with tabular or bar chart presentation rather than numerical aggregation across endpoints.	1) O'Bryan and Ross (1988) system
Endpoint scoring, with numerical aggregation	Numerical scoring of each endpoint assessed, with aggregation into either one overall score across all effects or a few scores representing the main effect types (e.g., human health, ecological, other environmental).	1) University of Tennessee (UT) Chemical Hazard Evaluation for Management Strategies (CHEMS-1) System (Swanson et al. 1997) 2) Informal Working Group on Priority Setting (IPS) (van der Zandt and van Leeuwen 1992) 3) Use Clusters Scoring System (UCSS) (USEPA 1993a)
Hybrid of endpoint scoring and decision rule approaches	Sorting chemicals into groups using pre-defined decision rules based on pre-defined criteria for some endpoints and scoring for other endpoints.	1) Accelerated Reduction Elimination of Toxics (ARET) System (Environment Canada and Ontario Ministry of Environment and Energy (OMOEE 1994) 2) Ontario "Bans, Phase-outs or Reductions" selection protocol (Socha et al. 1993) 3) Reportable Quantities (RQs) Method (USEPA 1989c)
Generic risk calculation	Simple risk calculation (e.g., exposure indicator ÷ toxicity indicator, with both in units of mg/kg-d) based on a "unit world" approach or a generic exposure scenario and default exposure modeling assumptions; results typically indexed rather than presented as risks.	1) Organization for Economic Cooperation and Development/ Screening Information Data Set (OECD/SIDS) (Auer 1992) 2) Toxic Release Inventory (TRI) Indicators Method (Bouwes and Hassur 1997)

Uses of chemical ranking and scoring systems

Chemical ranking and scoring systems have been created over the years by governments, academic institutions, and industry. For the most part, ranking and scoring systems are used for rapid assessment of the relative level of concern for individual chemicals within a group of chemicals. They usually consider the toxic effects of chemicals and some measure of exposure potential but typically are not intended to serve the same purpose as a QRA. Ranking and scoring systems have been applied in a variety of ways. Three broad types of uses include regulatory action, priority setting, and impact evaluation.

Chemical ranking and scoring systems can be used by different groups for a variety of purposes, as outlined below.

Government:
- Screen chemicals for further risk assessment or risk management.
- Screen chemical uses and industrial sectors for targeting risk reduction activities, including voluntary agreements and regulatory activities.
- Identify data gaps and chemical testing needs.
- Inform the regulated community about government priorities to encourage pollution prevention activities.
- Communicate relative hazard and exposure information to chemical manufacturers/users.
- Assist in risk-based allocation of resources.

Business:
- Determine data needs.
- Evaluate emissions for risk management actions for the local and global communities.
- Determine acceptability of existing and proposed new products.
- Provide input into corporate research and development activities.
- Provide input into changing product portfolios.
- Assist in product stewardship efforts, such as the Chemical Manufacturer's Association's Responsible Care Program.
- Assist in competitive analysis of products.
- Provide a basis for product selection by chemical users.

Environmental Organizations:
- Assist in choosing priorities for source/release reduction projects.
- Allow for participation in selection of chemicals for public reporting of chemical releases and transfers by facilities.
- Participate in decisions on which chemicals are persistent, bioaccumulative, and toxic (PBT) and should be candidates for phaseout.

Community Groups:
- Facilitate communication of potential chemical risk.
- Assist in product choice.
- Provide a basis for negotiations during development of community action plans.

Media:
- Assist in clear communication of relative potential risks and risk management activities.

Examples of some of the uses of ranking and scoring systems are discussed in the next section.

Direct regulatory/risk management action

Government resources are finite and must be used in such a way as to maximize the utility of public funds. The need for a more open and transparent basis for managing chemicals of concern has been a driving force behind the development of many CRS systems. Examples of this application are described below.

- The Comprehensive Environmental Response, Compensation and Liability Act (CERCLA) Section 102 Reportable Quantity Ranking Process (EMS 1985; USEPA 1989c) established reportable quantities (RQs) through a ranking process that takes into account environmental and human health hazards of chemicals on the CERCLA list. Reportable quantities are threshold quantities ranging from 1 to 5,000 lbs., above which certain chemical releases must be reported to the U.S. Environmental Protection Agency (USEPA).
- The Michigan Critical Materials Register (MCMR) (Michigan Department of Natural Resources [MDNR] 1987) ranking process results in a list of chemicals that may threaten water quality in Michigan. Chemicals included in the register are considered to pose a high degree of environmental concern, and companies must report their use and discharge of these chemicals.
- The Ontario Ministry of the Environment Scoring System (OMOE 1990) was used to generate the Ontario Effluent Monitoring Priority Pollutants List (EMPPL), a list of chemicals of environmental health concern that may threaten surface water quality in Ontario. Facilities belonging to 8 defined industrial sectors must report their discharge of listed chemicals. Discharge-limit regulations have been promulgated for each sector based on the monitoring of listed substances.
- The George Washington University (GWU) scoring system (Foran and Glenn 1993) was developed by nongovernmental organizations to serve as a tool for pollution prevention in the Great Lakes region through the identification of chemical substances for "sunsetting" (bans or phaseouts) and other regulatory or risk management activities.

Priority setting for further investigation

Several ranking and scoring systems have been developed specifically for assessing potential chemical hazards and risks for priority setting for regulatory and nonregulatory purposes. These purposes have included government/private sector partnerships for risk reduction, industry product stewardship programs, chemical management systems, and decisions on allocation of resources by government or industry.

*   The ITC Chemical Scoring System, developed by the Toxic Substances Control Act (TSCA) Interagency Testing Committee (ITC) in 1977, was the first system for the U.S. government to score and rank chemicals. The TSCA of 1976 created the ITC as an independent advisory committee to the administrator of the USEPA and gave the ITC responsibility for developing a system to evaluate, score, and rank chemicals for priority consideration by the administrator (Walker 1993a). Subsequent exercises were conducted in 1978, 1979, 1981, and 1983 (Walker 1993b, 1995). These systems, which all used sequential scoring for exposures followed by biological effects, are the only ones developed by affected parties, subjected to peer review through solicitations for public comments in the *Federal Register*, and modified to reflect the public comments. The ITC's chemical scoring exercises provided the initial catalyst for many of the CRS systems described in this book.

*   The Informal Working Group on Priority Setting (IPS) ranking method (van der Zandt and van Leeuwen 1992) was originally developed by a working group of European experts and further developed by the European Commission (EC) in collaboration with European Union (EU) member countries, industry, and nongovernmental organizations. The purpose of the IPS is to rank high-production-volume chemicals as a basis for selecting priority substances for risk assessment and risk management.

*   The Use Cluster Scoring System (UCSS) (USEPA 1993a) is aimed at measuring potential health and environmental concerns of chemicals that are used in industry clusters (i.e., certain common industrial uses) as a way of allocating resources for risk management. The relative concern scores are also provided to industry as a means of considering alternative chemicals and technologies.

*   The DuPont Product Stewardship Risk Characterization and Risk Management Guideline (Haaf 1995, 1997) uses measures of environmental and human health hazard to classify products into 3 categories. These categories are then used to determine the frequency of formal product stewardship reviews (2, 3, or 4 years) for chemicals and products.

*   The DuPont Engineering Standard on Occupational Health Priorities (Haaf 1995, 1997) uses chemical hazard and potential exposure as a means to assist industrial hygienists in assigning occupational priorities and risk management actions.

*   The Wet Milieugevaarlijke Stoffen (WMS) Scoring System (Könemann and Visser 1988; Timmer et al. 1988) was developed by the Directorate General for Environmental Protection of the Netherlands Ministry of Housing, Physical Planning,

and the Environment for use in industry, government, and academia for the selection of a limited number of chemicals as priorities for further investigation.

- The Agency for Toxic Substances and Disease Registry (ATSDR) System (ATSDR 1992) was created as a result of the U.S. Superfund Amendments and Reauthorization Act (SARA) of 1986, which required the ATSDR to prepare a list, in order of priority, of the hazardous substances commonly found at National Priority List (NPL) sites that pose the most significant potential human health threats. Substances on this priority list become candidates for the preparation of detailed toxicological profile reports prepared by ATSDR.

- The University of Tennessee (UT) Chemical Hazard Evaluation for Management Strategies (CHEMS-1) system (Swanson et al. 1997) prioritizes chemicals for safe substitute assessments, which could include the use of safer chemical substances or technologies with fewer adverse impacts. The system has also been used for impact evaluation, as discussed below, and for scoring of Toxics Release Inventory (TRI) releases from chemical production facilities.

- The Accelerated Reduction/Elimination of Toxics (ARET) System (Environment Canada and OMOEE 1994) uses hazard data to develop a list of toxic substances slated for action under the ARET project. The substances were selected from the Chemical Evaluation Search and Retrieval System (CESARS) database, which lists substances found in the Great Lakes basin.

Impact evaluation

Other ranking and scoring systems have been developed to evaluate the potential impacts of chemical releases. Examples include the following:

- The TRI Environmental Indicators Methodology (Bouwes and Hassur 1997) evaluates TRI chemical releases on a site-specific basis and derives a value to indicate the impacts of those releases by all facilities and to each environmental medium. Annual calculations of the indicator numbers allow a comparison of potential TRI chemical impacts from year to year. This system's output includes TRI indicators for chronic impacts on human health and the environment. These indicators yield measures related to risk, although not any physically meaningful measure (e.g., statistical risk to an individual).

- The CHEMS-1 system (Swanson et al. 1997) was modified to allow a comparative assessment of the relative hazard or risk posed by aggregate TRI chemical releases and transfers from an entire state or from facilities (Kincaid and Bartmess 1993). The modified system was used to assess, on a relative basis, the potential impacts from chemical releases for the 5 states with greatest releases (Tennessee, Texas, Louisiana, Indiana, and Ohio) and has also been used to score TRI releases from chemical production facilities.

Applicability to life-cycle assessment

Much attention has been focused on the methodology of LCA as a holistic approach for evaluating the effects on the environment associated with products, processes, or activities (Fava et al. 1993). A full LCA includes a quantitative inventory of resource and energy inputs and pollutant outputs and some form of impact assessment and improvement assessment. A life-cycle impact assessment is a process for assessing the potential and actual effects of environmental loadings identified in the inventory (Fava et al. 1993). Chemical ranking and scoring could become an essential element in the development of tools for assessing the impacts to health and the environment from chemical releases throughout the life cycle of products.

Life-cycle assessment has several uses, although its uses are more limited if some form of impact assessment is not included. Life-cycle assessment can be used for internal product improvements, designing new products, setting public policy on products and materials, and environmental labeling. Clearly, the different uses of LCA create different needs for impact assessment. An LCA used for internal product improvement, for example, might simply use the inventory component and operate on a "less-is-best" approach. An LCA used for setting public policy on materials or products would need to include some framework for assessing and comparing the significance of environmental releases and resource and energy use of the different products and materials being compared.

Life-cycle assessment and Design for the Environment are similar, but they do differ in several important ways. One major difference is in the focus of the effort. Design-for-the-Environment is a process by which consideration of pollution prevention is incorporated during the initial design of products and processes. However, during initial design, there is a need to make critical decisions, often with incomplete data, which will lead to an environmentally preferred product. In a sense, it is a process of constantly managing the material content and material use in a product. A CRS system may help in designing a product that minimizes the content of toxic materials.

Examples of systems that use CRS along with LCA include the following:

- The Environmental Priority Strategies (EPS) Enviro-Accounting Method (Steen and Ryding 1992) was developed to assess the health and ecological effects associated with the entire life cycle of a product, process, or activity. The main objective of the EPS method is to provide one overall economic measure of resource depletion and potential health and environmental impacts throughout a life cycle. In this system, values are assigned to impacts on the environment in terms of 5 "safeguard subjects" (human health, biodiversity, production, resources, and aesthetic values) according to willingness to pay to restore them to normal status. Chemical emissions (and other inventoried items) are then valued according to their estimated contribution to the changes in these safeguard subjects. The information on pollutant emissions originates from LCA-based inventory of the materials/process under study.

- The Motorola System (Hoffman 1997) is used in several ways and with differing levels of data intensity. All of the levels use a practical LCA process, which includes the stages of part/material sourcing, manufacturing, transportation, use, and end-of-life in order to assist the designer in making decisions that can have reduced environmental impacts in these stages.

Applications of chemical ranking and scoring systems

This section describes 7 CRS systems in more detail, with a discussion of their applications.

The Informal Working Group on Priority Setting System

The EU's Informal Working Group on Priority Setting (IPS) developed a chemical scoring system for use in the implementation of European Council Regulation EEC/793/93, which sets out a framework for evaluation and control of existing high-production-volume chemicals (Hansen 1993). Producers and importers of high-production-volume chemicals are required to submit data on specified human health and environmental endpoints and physical–chemical properties to the European Joint Research in Ispra, Italy, in a standard electronic format called the Harmonized Electronic Data Set (HEDSET). These data are loaded into the International Uniform Chemical Information Database (IUCLID) (Heidorn et al. 1996) and are scored and ranked by the IPS system. The IPS ranking system is intended to serve as a basis for choosing substances that will undergo an extensive risk assessment.

The IPS System is a consensus model by the developers of 4 CRS models used in 3 EU member states and in industry. When completed in 1992, the report and recommendations were presented for comments by the member state governments, industry, and nongovernmental organizations. A commission proposal was then prepared based on the comments received and discussed at 2 full technical meetings in 1993. The final IPS method was agreed upon at the second meeting with the agreement that discussion on the method could be reopened at a later date when more experience had been gained in the use of the method.

The IUCLID–IPS interface contains built-in data selection preferences, so that generally the most "conservative" test result within the preferred test for the endpoint is selected. For human health, carcinogenicity, genetic toxicity, reproductive toxicity, respiratory sensitivity, repeated dose toxicity, acute toxicity, irritation, and skin sensitization, endpoint scores are combined into a human health effects score. A human exposure value is calculated based upon the percentage of the substance to which humans are estimated to be exposed and the tonnage produced. Aquatic toxicity data are used to represent ecotoxicity in the model. Data gaps are filled by the use of structure-activity relationships (SARs) and expert judgment.

Accelerated Reduction/Elimination of Toxics

The objective of the ARET project is to achieve the elimination of, or significant reduction in, emissions of specific toxic substances from Canadian sources through voluntary efforts (Environment Canada and OMOEE 1994). The project focuses on persistent, bioaccumulative, and toxic substances, although reductions in release of other toxic substances are also recognized. ARET is steered by a multistakeholder committee with members drawn from the Canadian federal government, provincial governments, industry associations, and professional associations. ARET was initiated by Environment Canada, and that agency continues to provide the steering committee with a Secretariat through the National Office of Pollution Prevention.

Central to the ARET project is the ARET Candidate Substances List, which is subdivided into several component lists. The lists were generated through the application of a scoring/screening system. The ARET substance selection system is an adaptation of the system developed by the OMOEE and used in its municipal–industrial strategy for abatement (MISA), surface water monitoring program (OMOE 1990) and the "Candidate Substances List for Bans, Phase-Outs or Reductions" project (Socha et al. 1993). Modifications were made according to the recommendations of a multistakeholder subcommittee composed of representatives of government, industry, environmental groups, and labor.

In the ARET system, scores are assigned to a set of parameters including persistence, bioaccumulation potential, and toxicity (acute lethality; chronic/subchronic toxicity to mammals, non-mammals, and plants; teratogenicity; and carcinogenicity). Approximately 500 substances found in the ambient environment or known to be emitted in Canada were screened through the ARET system. Substances receiving high scores for all 3 selection criteria (persistence, bioaccumulation, and toxicity) were placed on ARET List A. Other toxic substances were placed on ARET List B. The lists may be further subdivided as shown in Table 1-2.

Table 1-2 ARET substance lists

List	Criteria met or exceeded	Goal
A-1	Persistent, bioaccumulative, and toxic (PBT)	Elimination in long term, significant reduction in short term
A-2	As with A-1, but consensus on evaluation was not achieved among all stakeholders	
B-1	Persistent and toxic	Reduced emission
B-2	Bioaccumulative and toxic	Reduced emission
B-3	Toxic	Reduced emission

Participation in ARET is voluntary. Participants are asked to submit an inventory of emissions of candidate substances and an action plan for substance emission elimination and/or reduction in the short term. Annual reports on participation and progress will be issued by the ARET Secretariat.

Use Cluster Scoring System

The TSCA allows the USEPA to regulate chemicals or chemical mixtures that present or will present an unreasonable risk of injury to health or the environment. Within USEPA, the provisions of TSCA are implemented by the Office of Pollution Prevention and Toxics (OPPT, formerly the Office of Toxic Substances). As of 1995, there are over 70,000 chemicals on the TSCA inventory, of which 15,000 are non-polymeric substances with production volumes greater than 10,000 lbs. per year (U.S. Congress 1995). Historically, OPPT has approached the evaluation of this large number of existing chemicals by choosing chemicals to evaluate based on receipt of new hazard data from the manufacturer; at the request of other USEPA offices, government agencies, or interested parties; or by targeting specific sets of chemicals, like those listed on the TRI or chemicals that are persistent and bioaccumulative. While this approach created a manageable set of chemicals to evaluate, it has not comprehensively addressed potential toxicity issues.

The UCSS (USEPA 1993a) was created as one tool to systematically identify and screen concerns related to a greater number of chemicals in commerce. The UCSS is currently being used in the USEPA's Design for the Environment Program (USEPA 1995c) as a means of selecting processes within industrial production systems that are priorities for Cleaner Technologies Substitutes Assessments (Kincaid et al. 1996).

A use cluster is a set of chemicals and technologies that may potentially substitute for each other in a particular use. The UCSS uses easily obtainable information on hazard and exposure to rank and score chemicals as defined by use. The system is designed as a screening mechanism to rank individual chemicals within clusters and then use these scores to rank the clusters into high, medium, and low concern categories. The system provides a measure of potential risk based on readily available information, although it is not intended to be a substitute for a detailed risk assessment.

The system generates a score that gives a sense of the potential concerns and relative significance associated with a group of chemicals used in similar applications. Six components are combined to produce the overall UCSS score. Two components measure potential contact with a chemical or physical agent (potential human exposure and potential ecological exposure), and two measure inherent toxicological properties of a chemical (potential human hazard and potential ecological hazard). The potential human exposure and potential human hazard are ranked separately and then multiplied to yield a potential human risk score. Similarly, the potential ecological exposure and potential ecological hazard are scored and combined to produce a potential ecological risk score. These 2 indicator scores are then summed with the fifth component, an indicator of past USEPA interest for each cluster chemical. The mean of this value for all the chemicals in a cluster is summed with the sixth component, an indicator of the cluster's potential for reduction of concern through pollution prevention (pollution prevention potential score) to arrive at the final overall cluster score. (*Editor's note:* In a later version of this system, the pollution prevention potential and USEPA interest scores were taken out of the initial screening procedure but retained as options for final cluster selection by system users [F. Hall 1996 personal communication].)

The Michigan Critical Materials Register

The Michigan Critical Materials Register (MCMR) is a list of chemicals of high environmental concern from a water pollution perspective (MDNR 1987). Every business within Michigan using the critical materials must file an annual report of their use, discharge, and/or disposal of these chemicals. Candidates for MCMR consideration come from various lists of environmental contaminants and potential problem chemicals. A chemical is selected for placement on the register only after extensive literature review defining its adverse effects and then scoring via a detailed hazard assessment process. This methodology considers acute toxicity, carcinogenicity, mutagenicity, reproductive and developmental effects, bioaccumulation, other toxicity (including subacute and chronic toxicity and phytotoxicity) as well as physical–chemical properties and environmental fate. Chemicals are scored as to their level of concern, and those posing a high environmental concern are included on the register.

The Interagency Testing Committee systems

The ITC conducted a series of 6 scoring exercises from 1977 to 1987 to develop CRS systems that were used to evaluate chemicals for priority consideration by the USEPA Administrator. Each exercise consisted of a workshop attended by representatives from federal, state, industry, academic, and public interest groups. Representatives were selected for participation based on their expertise to evaluate, score, and rank chemicals for potential exposures (occupational, consumer, general population, or environmental), for potential to persist or bioaccumulate, for potential to cause ecological effects (wildlife, aquatic organisms, or terrestrial plants), or for potential to cause health effects (acute, subchronic, reproductive, developmental, mutagenic, or oncogenic). The exposure, persistence, or bioaccumulation potential factors and criteria developed by the ITC to score and rank chemicals include annual production volume, occupational exposure, consumer exposure, persistence, and bioaccumulation. The biological effects include acute toxicity, subchronic toxicity, mutagenicity, carcinogenicity, developmental toxicity, and aquatic toxicity. These factors are used by USEPA's new and existing chemical programs and others to score and rank chemicals.

Values for some of the biological effects can be estimated using quantitative structure-activity relationships (QSAR) and other biological effects models. This includes the Substructure-based Computerized Chemical Selection Expert System (SuCCSES), developed as part of the sixth scoring exercise to identify groups of chemicals that share the same chemical substructure and the potential to cause the same health or ecological effect (Walker and Brink 1989; Walker 1991, 1995). Data on biological effects can be obtained by adding a chemical to the ITC's Priority Testing List. In addition to these data, SuCCSES can be used to identify chemicals that have the potential to cause similar effects based on a common substructure or to identify chemicals that do not share a common substructure but that do share the potential to cause a common biological effect.

Republic of Korea's chemical ranking and scoring approach

The Republic of Korea's Ministry of Environment is developing a CRS system as a step toward expanding the existing environmental quality standards. The demand for environmental protection is relatively high. The government is coping with this demand by implementing existing environmental laws or regulations. In the process, environmental quality standards are one of the most important points of concern. Generally, the number of chemicals regulated by environmental quality standards is lower than the number regulated in more developed countries. The public feels unsafe with the imbalance. The government is under pressure to increase the number of standards with a rational and, if possible, economical approach. The ultimate solution of selecting chemicals needing standards should come from comprehensive risk assessment; however, CRS could be a good starting point. This approach should be beneficial to other developing countries as well.

USEPA's Waste Minimization Prioritization Tool

USEPA's Office of Solid Waste (OSW) established a partnership with OPPT in fall 1996 to develop a chemical risk screening tool to assist OSW and other stakeholders in identifying waste minimization priorities (USEPA 1997a). This tool, the Waste Minimization Prioritization Tool (WMPT), was developed in conjunction with the Waste Minimization National Plan, which established goals for reducing the most persistent, bioaccumulative, and toxic chemicals in the nation's hazardous wastes (USEPA 1994a). The WMPT is derived from, and shares much in common with, OPPT's UCSS.

The WMPT provides a means of conducting initial risk screening of chemicals in wastes based on their persistence, bioaccumulation potential, chronic human and ecological toxicity, and quantity (mass). OSW plans to use the WMPT to identify chemicals of concern at a national level for the purpose of tracking progress toward the goals of the Waste Minimization National Plan. The relative chemical rankings derived from the WMPT can also be used by other stakeholders to identify waste minimization priorities. For example, USEPA, regions, and states, in directing their waste minimization implementation efforts, can mesh the national chemicals of concern with other chemicals that are a regional or state priority and identify waste streams likely to contain them. In addition, OSW plans to make the WMPT and chemical rankings derived from it available to waste generators, trade associations, and others to support their waste minimization efforts.

Data and Databases for Chemical Ranking and Scoring

Collecting the data needed to score and rank a substance is typically the most expensive and time-consuming part of CRS. Most of the CRS systems that have been developed have created their own database of hazard and exposure parameters for the list of chemicals to be evaluated. This has resulted in duplication of effort because few of the databases have been readily accessible to other developers and users of CRS systems.

Toward a common, chemical-specific database

If data were collected and organized in a specific format, they could be made accessible to other users of CRS systems. A database of intrinsic physical–chemical and toxicological data would be helpful to users of CRS systems, and a companion database of extrinsic exposure-related information (e.g., production, use, and release volumes) would be useful for comparing exposure situations in various regions to each other or to a region of interest. The latter would also be useful in integrating local exposure information to derive regional, national, or international scores. Should a common, accessible database be developed, data quality assurance issues would need to be addressed and agreed upon.

Three precedents exist for harmonized databases of chemical information. The Chemical Evaluation Search & Retrieval System (CESARS) is a text-oriented database originated by the MDNR and currently maintained and updated by MDNR and the OMOEE. CESARS contains data for approximately 1,000 substances and is available on-line. TOM-CAT (OMOEE 1994) is a database containing the "Ontario Environmental Assessments" components of CESARS, including OMOEE/ARET scores. This is a relational database and is searchable using various query structures. TOMCAT is also used as a data-entry tool and can generate standard-format text files for inclusion in CESARS. TOMCAT contains data for approximately 700 substances and is currently available only to OMOEE, Environment Canada, Health Canada, and the ARET Secretariat. The IUCLID is Oracle-based and is a multilingual (currently the original 9 EU languages), glossary-based database which contains the data on the EU high-production-volume chemicals that have been submitted by industry following Council Regulation EEC/793/93. The IUCLID database software is copyrighted by the EC and is available through the European Chemicals Bureau (ECB) at cost recovery for the installation. The IUCLID has been or is being installed at the 15 EU member states (with multiple installations in some member states), approximately 40 European companies, the OECD secretariat in Paris, the International Registry of Potentially Toxic Chemicals (IRPTC) in Geneva, the USEPA in Washington, and Japan. Most of these data are nonconfidential, including the physical–chemical properties, chemical fate and pathways, and ecotoxicity and toxicity data. The nonconfidential data have been made available on a compact disk (CD-ROM) as a stand-alone database of chemical profiles.

With regard to use, release, and production databases, the OECD is working toward the establishment of a standardized international format for pollutant transfer and release registries (PTRRs). To avoid loss of information, critical data used for scoring should be highlighted in a common database, e.g., as a separate searchable field.

Handling data gaps

Frequently, no data exist for a given property or endpoint for a particular substance. The CRS system must be able to cope with such "data gaps." It is generally preferable to fill data gaps in a data-neutral manner. Possible approaches include these:

- Use of an alternative surrogate endpoint for scoring purposes. For example, the ARET system assigns a score for genotoxicity/mutagenicity in the absence of carcinogenicity data, and the USEPA Hazard Ranking System (HRS) uses acute mammalian toxicity data to evaluate chronic toxicity if chronic toxicity data are unavailable.
- Application of QSAR or SAR where possible and appropriate. The models employed must be well-accepted as adequately predictive. QSAR/SAR-derived data are generally used the same way as data derived from laboratory and field studies, i.e., no additional "safety factors" are applied.
- Assignment of an empirically derived default value for the score (e.g., the median or geometric mean of the scores assigned to other substances for the same endpoint).
- Postponing evaluation or scoring of a chemical until data are developed.
- Sensitivity analysis to determine the impact of the data gap on the overall score and rank if no measured data are readily available and no acceptable QSAR estimate can be applied.
- Expert evaluation of the chemicals. For example, in the absence of data, the ITC Scoring System assigns scores based upon expert evaluation for the various biological effects.

Assignment of high-score or low-score defaults results in penalizing or rewarding substances where data gaps exist. This approach should be applied with an awareness of its tendency to drive the results. In most cases, a data-neutral approach to handling data gaps is preferable. There may be some instances, however, when data gaps are handled in a biased manner because of the system's intended use. It should be noted that it is not necessarily conservative to assign a maximum default value for missing data because this can lead to higher ranks for chemicals without any data as compared to those with ample data demonstrating a moderate-to-high hazard.

Handling of data gaps is discussed in detail in Chapters 2 through 5, dealing with specific hazard endpoints and exposure-related parameters.

Tracking data gaps

One of the benefits of a CRS system is the highlighting of specific data deficits. This information (i.e., where data are deficient) can be included within the scoring system, the associated database, and the system's output. "Flags" within the scoring system output or the database indicate those substances requiring further research and indicating the types of research required (e.g., toxicity testing, generation of monitoring, and exposure data).

Ranking and Scoring Chemical Mixtures

The assessment of mixtures of substances can be complex, in particular when the individual components of a mixture are not closely related chemically or toxicologically. The investigation of potential additive, antagonistic, and synergistic effects of substances when exposure is to a mixture is an important research need.

For the purpose of CRS, the practical approach in most instances is to evaluate the component substances of a mixture individually. Exceptions to this include the following:

- When data are available from studies performed using the mixture itself, it may be practical to evaluate the mixture as a whole. This is often the case when the mixture is composed of related substances (e.g., toxaphene, polychlorinated biphenyl [PCB] mixtures, and distillation fractions such as gasoline, light petroleum distillates, or solvent naphtha). The USEPA MIXTOX database compiles existing data on the toxicological effects of some mixtures (USEPA 1992d).

- When the mixture is composed of isomers of a substance with comparable physical–chemical and toxicological properties (e.g., xylene, which may be a mixture of o-, m-, and p-isomers, or toluene diisocyanate, which may be a mixture of 2 isomers), the user could evaluate the isomers individually and assign final "mixture" scores by using the highest score among the isomers for each scoring element.

Note that when exposure is being evaluated, the relative proportion of individual component substances in a mixture may become important, particularly if those components have dissimilar properties. Those proportions may not remain constant for a given named mixture, e.g., solvent naphtha, creosote, or waste stream types.

Scaling, Aggregation, Weighting, and Decision Theory

Chemical ranking and scoring systems typically utilize data on several different health and environmental endpoints and score these data on a common scale or use decision rules so that the data can be combined and compared for each chemical. Often, scores for different toxicological endpoints are aggregated within endpoint categories (e.g., chronic human health) and aggregated across human health and environmental impact categories to yield one score that combines all categories for each chemical. In aggregating across impact categories, an explicit or implicit weight is often assigned to each category based upon some consideration of the relative importance of each category to the decision-maker. Complex formal decision systems can be used to combine disparate data to yield one result for the decision-maker, but most systems in use rely upon pragmatic and simple methods. The results of a CRS can be highly influenced by the manner in which data on each chemical are scored, scaled, aggregated, and weighted. While no system's results can be independent of the methodology used to interpret and combine the data, the practitioner should describe clearly the operations performed on the data, should have some basis in theory for these operations, and should be aware of and communicate their influence on the results.

Scaling

Scaling occurs when the raw data on chemical toxicity or physical–chemical properties are translated to some type of numeric or qualitative scale. For instance, ranges of values of LD50 for acute rodent toxicity can be assigned numbers (1, 2, 3) or high, medium, and low designations. This type of scale is called an "ordinal scale," where all that can be said about the numbers or designations is that one is higher or lower than the others. Some data are expressed in simple "yes" or "no" (or "1" or "0") terms, such as whether a particular chemical is a skin sensitizer or not. This type of scale is called a "nominal scale."

Actual data may be used for the scoring so that the scale has some physical significance. Where the particular scale upon which these numbers are placed has no natural zero, as with commonly used temperature scales, this type of scale is called an "interval scale." With the Celsius scale, for instance, the difference between a temperature of 20° and 40° is the same as the difference between 40° and 60°, but one cannot say that 40° is twice as hot as 20°. Finally, where the particular scale upon which the numbers are placed naturally passes through zero, such as with density or vapor pressure (Pv), the scale is called a "ratio scale."

Aggregation and weighting

Many CRS systems in use score health and environmental endpoints on ordinal scales (1, 2, 3 or high, medium, low), as described above, and perform simple mathematical operations to combine the scores for different endpoints and different impact categories. Mathematical operations performed using ordinal scales do not yield results that have any more meaning mathematically than the individual scales themselves. Adding a "3" score to a "2" score may yield a "5", but the interval between "5" and "4" is not the same as the interval between "4" and "3", nor is "4" twice as toxic as "2". All that can be said is that a chemical with two "3" scores is relatively more toxic than a chemical with a "3" and a "2" (where "1" is lower than "2" and "3").

These mathematical operations often bring in weighting to express the relative importance of one health or environmental endpoint or impact category as compared to others. Where scores are aggregated by addition, weighting is often applied as a multiplier to each score (e.g., $w_1 S_1 + w_2 S_2$, etc.). Weighting appears at each aggregation step, whether it is implicit or explicit. For example, if all scores are aggregated without any weighting factors or multipliers, then an implicit equal weighting has been performed. (It should be noted that numerical aggregation could give more credibility to summary numbers than appropriate, implying a precision or accuracy that does not exist. One alternative is to report results in categories rather than actual summary scores, e.g., 1 to 20 = very low, 21 to 40 = low, 41 to 60 = moderate, 61 to 80 = high, 81 to 100 = very high.)

An approach often used that avoids performing mathematical operations on ordinal scale scores is to apply simple decision rules. For instance, some systems rank a chemical "high" if it ranks high in any one health or environmental endpoint score. Others use the most sensitive health and environmental endpoint for a chemical to represent the overall relative risk of the chemical on the theory that this health or environmental effect will be experienced before higher levels of exposure give rise to other effects. Still others take a matrix approach (e.g., Table 1-3), which combines scores in such a way as to weight the results toward the higher of the two scores.

Table 1-3 Result scores for aggregation of high, medium, and low scores

	High	Medium	Low
High	High	High	High
Medium	High	Medium	Medium
Low	High	Medium	Low

Given that aggregation and weighting are frequently used in CRS systems, it is an important research need to examine in more detail how they are performed and how the methods can be made more consistent and transparent. It should be clear that scientific judgment is involved in the scoring of endpoint data (such as the ranges that are considered high, medium, or low), and it is possible to evolve a scientific consensus on such scoring for most health and environmental endpoints. What is not so clear is how scientific judgment and some scientific consensus-building processes can be brought to bear upon aggregation and weighting issues because aggregation and weighting methods have not been considered scientific issues.

Because of the lack of transparency and inconsistencies introduced by scaling, aggregation, and weighting, it is understandable that some practitioners advocate presenting only raw data or presenting scores without any aggregation. It is impossible to avoid aggregation and weighting, however, by simply not formalizing the process. Even if the endpoints are not aggregated by the practitioner, the user of the results likely will aggregate to make risk management decisions.

Decision analysis or decision theory

More formal methods exist for decision-making where there are multiple criteria or attributes that must be assessed at the same time. Decision analysis is a technique for selecting among options available to a decision-maker in a logical framework. Formal decision analysis methods include Multi-Attribute Utility Theory and the Analytic Hierarchy Process (Saaty 1980). A detailed discussion of these formal methods is beyond the scope of this report, and they have rarely been used in CRS systems. In Multi-Attribute Utility Theory, the relative importance of each of the attributes to the overall decision is assessed, and a utility function is developed for each. In the Analytic Hierarchy Process, paired comparisons between each attribute in the system are used to derive an overall weighting of all attributes.

Presentation and Communication of CRS Results

Presentation and communication are vital elements of CRS. Without effective communication to decision-makers, CRS will not contribute to improving environmental performance. Reporting should be objective and transparent, and there should be a clear indication of what has and what has not been included in the study. Any assumptions that were made should be clearly listed and explained.

The needs of different audiences should be recognized and addressed when the study is presented or disseminated. Target audiences can include companies, trade associations, government agencies, environmental groups, scientific/technical communities, and other nongovernmental organizations (e.g., consumers). Communication in the public domain is especially critical because the risks of misinterpretation are heightened when CRS-derived information is provided to audiences not familiar with the complexities of risk ranking and risk management.

Good reporting and communication practice start at the outset of the CRS. Relevant project details and all data should be obtained and compiled in a way that allows subsequent access, manipulation, and if necessary, scrutiny. Once the CRS has been completed and all the data processed, the next stage, ideally, is the production of a complete report.

A complete report should contain tables of data and should ensure transparency and consistency of all the methodologies and data employed. The report should constitute the primary input to the scientific/technical audience and should provide a base from which summary reports to other target audiences could be prepared. These later summaries should be tailored to the recipient requirements, should be labeled as summaries only, and should include appropriate reference to the primary report and data sources to ensure that they are not taken out of context.

Goals and scope of the study

The presentation or communication of any CRS should include a clear and concise statement of the overall goals of the analysis. The degree of analysis and resulting documentation will vary, depending on these differing goals, and it is recognized that the depth of documentation increases with any external use of the CRS report.

The scope of the study is directly linked to the goals and potential uses of the study results. The rationale for choosing the amount and type of toxicological and exposure data should be described.

Methodology

A full description of the methodology used for a particular CRS should be presented. This includes the method of ranking and scoring and the types of prescreens and tiers used. It is recognized that the various current methodologies may be data limited, and thus, calculations, estimates, or extrapolations may be used, all of which may influence the overall results. Chemical ranking and scoring reports should explicitly identify when SAR models are used to fill data gaps and when professional judgments are used.

Data sources

The data used in CRS systems come from a wide range of sources, which can be of widely differing quality. All such issues should be addressed in the report. Any private data used in a public study, but not disclosed, should be clearly noted. The sources of all public data (e.g., databases, specifically referenced textbooks, government reports, or previous CRS systems) should be clearly identified.

Key indicators of data selection criteria should also be reported. Some selection criteria are as follows:
- geographic scope (site-specific versus industry-averaged);
- time-period covered (points collected for one week, one year, etc.);
- completeness (missing or partial data, data gaps);
- representativeness (degree to which data represent the population);
- accuracy;
- uncertainty (lack of consistency; use of estimates from different processes — similar, more easily measured — or of nondetectable limits); and
- surrogate species.

The report should describe how uncertainty in data and methods may influence the results of the analysis. Major sources of uncertainty, the magnitude of the uncertainty, and the potential influence of the uncertainty on the final results should be addressed. Sensitivity analyses are strongly encouraged.

Data presentation

Depending on end use, data should be presented in full detail in the report, utilizing simplifications only when necessary or when protecting proprietary data. It is often appropriate to present the data in the form of histograms, spreadsheets, grids, etc., to facilitate interpretation. There should be a complete reference to all data sources, or the data should be available upon request. Presentation of the ranking itself should include the chemical identification (e.g., name, Chemical Abstracts Service [CAS] Registry number) and any information required to make the ranking transparent.

Conclusions

Any conclusions drawn from the study should be explicit, limited to chemicals or products actually examined, appropriate to the variability of the data used in the analyses, and wholly based on the results and methodologies presented in the report. Where additional materials are introduced to augment the conclusions or for purposes of comparison, appropriate reference should be made to their sources.

Implications derived from the conclusions can involve interpretation and thus may be subjective. Ideally, they should be based solely on conclusions of the study and incorporate an explicit explanation of subjective judgments.

Summary

The report should contain an appropriate summary. The summary should stand alone without compromising the results of the CRS. The target audience of the report typically will be decision-makers who may not have sufficient time or background to read the full report. Therefore, the summary report also should fulfill the criteria for transparency, consistency, etc., as would the complete report. At a minimum, the summary report should include the goals and scope, and it should clearly indicate what is expected to be achieved by the screening.

Principles for Development and Selection of CRS Systems

This section presents and elaborates on a series of fundamental principles underlying the overall framework of CRS. These principles apply to the development of a system as well as to the selection of a system for a particular application. While desirable from the perspective of reducing confusion arising from a multiplicity of systems, no single CRS can meet all needs at this time. The elements of the CRS used and the way they are evaluated and combined may differ depending on the scope of evaluation and the specific application. That is, CRS used for different applications and levels of complexity may reasonably be expected to take different forms. Furthermore, given the large number of existing systems with overlapping objectives and the confusion this can cause, those with a need for a CRS should investigate the literature and carefully consider adopting an existing system rather than developing a new one. However, all CRS variants should be consistent with the general principles described below.

1) A CRS system should have a clearly defined purpose: It is critical that the purpose be defined and stated as precisely as possible, before a new CRS system is developed or an existing CRS system is selected for a specific application.

2) A CRS system should be compatible with the risk assessment paradigm: Chemical ranking systems should be, to the extent possible, consistent with the general risk assessment paradigm in which hazard and exposure are assessed and integrated into some expression of risk. Chemical ranking systems may actually employ the same methods as QRA. (This does not mean, however, that CRS is generally equivalent to risk assessment, and it should not be represented or applied as such.) Chemical ranking systems based on hazard or exposure alone may be appropriate for some applications.

3) Uncertainty should be acknowledged and assessed: A chemical ranking system is by definition highly uncertain, and applications should acknowledge and communicate the uncertainty in the results. Chemical ranking systems should not be used to make fine distinctions between chemicals, nor should it be the exclusive means to make decisions with major adverse impact or resource implications.

4) The role for professional judgment should be acknowledged: Professional judgment and qualitative assessment are appropriate, and in some cases necessary, within the context of CRS. It should not be considered mandatory, nor necessarily even desirable, to quantify all aspects of a CRS system. Professional judgment should be used routinely (e.g., in a confirmation step to "validate" the results of any CRS application).

5) There should be a broad consideration of effects: In ranking chemicals released to the environment, human health, ecological, and as appropriate to the specific application and goals, other environmental effects should be considered. In some applications, effects of both acute and chronic exposures should be considered. Ideally, fundamentally different effect types should be considered in separate subcomponents, or "modules," within a CRS system so that the toxicity and exposure measures relevant to each can be considered in the most appropriate manner.

6) The role of valuation in aggregation and weighting should be recognized: Numerical aggregation and weighting across broad effect types (e.g., human health versus ecological versus other environmental effects) and across endpoints within effect types (e.g., cancer versus noncancer effects) require value judgments that are not the exclusive domain of technical experts and need to incorporate input representing the public or a spectrum of decision-makers. Relative weighting of these diverse effect types is dependent on the risk management context and should be determined on a situation-specific basis. Therefore, it generally is preferable that a chemical ranking system not aggregate across major effect types; if such aggregation is deemed necessary, the system should be transparent about

the tradeoffs incorporated and should present results in both aggregated and disaggregated form.

7) Methods and outputs should be transparent: The way a CRS system works should be understandable to practitioners in the field, and the system outputs should be explainable to decision-makers. As provided for in Principle 2, a CRS system should be based on an underlying theoretical logic consistent with the general risk assessment paradigm. That logic — including the logic for mathematical formulations — should be clearly explained and documented.

8) A CRS system should be neutral to data availability: In general, a CRS should not systematically "punish" or "reward" chemicals with extensive data versus chemicals with no data (e.g., minimum or maximum default scores should not be awarded based on missing data). In some cases, depending on the objective of the specific CRS application, a "non-neutral" approach may be appropriate. If the objective, for example, is to provide an incentive for data collection, it may be appropriate to treat certain data gaps in a non-neutral manner (e.g., give high scores). In any case, any bias in the method used to fill data gaps should be made explicit.

9) A CRS system should accommodate extreme variability in data availability across chemicals: Chemical ranking systems should recognize and attempt to accommodate the fact that chemicals have extremely variable hazard- and exposure-related databases. At the least, all systems must distinguish high-threat chemicals from chemicals with missing data.

10) A tiered approach is practical and desirable: For reasons of practicality and cost-effectiveness, tiers (levels) of increasing CRS complexity and/or data requirements are desirable. The appropriate tier should be determined by the scope of the application (e.g., number of chemicals, amount of data needed, site-specific versus national decision-making), the possible outcome of the application (e.g., risk management action versus ranking for more data collection), and the resources available. A CRS should be only as complex and data-intensive as absolutely necessary to meet the objective of the specific application. As a general guideline, simpler is better with regard to CRS design.

11) Similar effects/exposure categories should be assessed across tiers: Ideally, initial tiers should be based on the same effects and exposure categories used in succeeding tiers but should incorporate them in a simpler and less data-intensive way. For example, if toxicity and exposure are both part of the final tier, then the initial tier should include both considerations as well. If the initial tier, however, is based on toxicity or exposure alone, then some mechanism to identify significant false negatives/positives should be included.

12) Critical information should be preserved: Chemical ranking and scoring outputs should preserve critical information about chemicals in an organized and readily available format so that they are easy to verify and/or use in alternative ranking procedures. When CRS outputs are single scores, a system of flags or codes

should be considered to transmit critical information (e.g., indicators of data gaps, data quality, and significant effects that drive scores).

13) Data selection guidelines should be specified: Guidelines for data selection, including acceptable data sources, data source hierarchies, and other data selection and manipulation rules, should be fully and precisely specified to ensure that the most appropriate data inputs are used for each chemical.

14) A CRS system should be theory driven as well as data driven: While data availability is clearly an important consideration in CRS development, an underlying theoretical logic should be developed first and then meshed with data availability considerations.

15) Sensitivity analysis should be performed: Sensitivity analysis is an important step in CRS development to examine how the spread of empirical data and the range of anticipated conditions affect the system outputs and to identify which system elements appear to be the main "drivers" of the results.

16) Pre-selection of chemicals should be consistent with the CRS: Any pre-selection of chemicals should be consistent with the CRS system being applied, or at a minimum, the impacts of the pre-selection approach should be examined. Because pre-selection is generally based on very simple factors, some type of flagging or double-checking to prevent significant false negatives is needed.

17) The impacts of scaling should be considered: In systems that assign numerical scores, there is a need to recognize scaling issues (e.g., whether a scale is ordinal, interval, or ratio) and how they affect aggregation. The kinds of scales in a system and the mathematics of combining values should be clearly described.

Recommendations

The differences between the numerous CRS systems should be resolved to the extent possible and should be consistent with the applications by attention to the principles elaborated in this document and by use of common databases. In order to make progress toward such a resolution, the following steps are recommended:

1) There should be better communication and coordination among CRS practitioners in international and U.S. organizations and also among U.S. state and federal agencies in utilizing these systems.

2) A common database of physical–chemical properties, intrinsic exposure-related data, and toxicological data should be developed for use by CRS practitioners.

3) Companies and trade associations should use CRS in carrying out product stewardship.

4) An inventory of CRS systems should be maintained in order to make best use of resources and to inform practitioners.

5) There should be a "round robin" demonstration of currently used CRS systems on the same chemical dataset to allow evaluation of the CRS systems' similarities and differences.

6) The Society of Environmental Toxicology and Chemistry (SETAC) should provide a forum for advancements in the field of CRS.

7) SETAC should conduct further workshops in the area of CRS, including workshops that focus on data selection guidance, generic risk assessment, and aggregation and weighting.

Chapter 2

Measures of Exposure

Mary Swanson, chapter editor
Robert S. Boethling, John Evans, John P. Geisy, James W. Gillett, Philip Howard, David
Jeffrey, Jay Jon, Preben Kristensen, Robert Larson, Yong-Hwa Kim

Characterizing human health and ecological risk from chemical releases to the environment requires some method to assess exposure. The amount of exposure depends on several factors, including the amount of chemical used or released, chemical fate and transport, chemical concentration at the point of exposure, the routes and rates of uptake, the exposure setting, and characteristics of receptors potentially exposed to the chemical. In quantitative risk assessment (QRA), these factors are typically combined to estimate a potential human dose rate and concentrations to which organisms in the environment are exposed.

Although chemical scoring systems vary widely in their complexity, they share a common scientific foundation derived from the paradigm of risk assessment. Chemical ranking and scoring (CRS) is similar to QRA in that evaluations of both chemical toxicity and exposure are incorporated in some way. However, the exposure assessment component of CRS is typically qualitative or semiquantitative at best. For large numbers of chemicals, a quantitative and site-specific estimate of exposure for each chemical would be too resource-intensive for practical purposes. Chemical ranking and scoring systems use a variety of surrogate parameters to estimate exposure (pounds or kilograms of a chemical released per year, for example).

Some of the issues initially identified by the Exposure Assessment Workgroup include the following:
- What is the state of the science?
- What are the different degrees of sophistication or complexity, and is a tiered approach appropriate?
- What level of uncertainty is acceptable for CRS?
- What are the possible purposes for CRS, and what type of exposure data would be required?
- How might the definition of exposure vary with the CRS application?
- What spatial and temporal considerations are relevant (e.g., site-specific versus generic exposure levels, time frame)?

- Should measures of exposure, in the context of CRS, be route- or media-specific?
- When (if ever) would using a "standard environment" (e.g., Mackay's [1991] unit world approach) be appropriate?
- How might the probability of exposures to a concentration be compared to effects?
- What are the relevant data issues, and what are the options (e.g., use of SARs, QSARs, use of predicted versus measured data).
- What is a minimum dataset for exposure in CRS?
- What research needs have been identified?
- What principles will enhance credibility (e.g., transparency) of exposure in CRS?

This chapter describes the state of the science for assessing exposure within the context of CRS and the different types of exposure measures that have been used in CRS. This is followed by a discussion of structure and tiers for the exposure component of CRS and a discussion of data issues. Finally, the working group's findings and recommendations are presented, concluding with a summary and recommendations for further work.

State of the Science

An exposure assessment is an evaluation of the contact an organism may have with a chemical or physical agent and describes the amount, frequency, duration, and route of contact. Guidance documents for QRA exposure assessment include the USEPA's Risk Assessment Guidance for Superfund (USEPA 1989b), Guidelines for Exposure Assessment (USEPA 1992a), and the Dermal Exposure Assessment Guidance (USEPA 1992b), which describe exposure assessment in detail. The reader is referred to these and the literature for more information.

There are several factors that affect potential exposure to a chemical. Types of exposure parameters or measures that have been used in various CRS systems include those listed below.

1) Chemical use or emission characteristics — i.e., the amount of chemical released, the release location and/or media. Data include the following:
   - production, use, and disposal (PUD) amounts (volume or mass);
   - market information; and
   - emission data.

2) Chemical properties — i.e., chemical transport, partitioning after release; chemical transformation/degradation. Data include the following:
   - chemical structure or composition;
   - basic physical–chemical properties; and

- properties related to chemical persistence and transformation, bioaccumulation, and mobility.

3) Estimated or measured chemical concentration. Data include the following:
   - measured environmental concentrations,
   - frequency of occurrence,
   - estimated environmental concentrations, and
   - sensitivity and accuracy of environmental measurements.

4) Exposure setting and/or receptor characteristics. This information includes the following:
   - location and number of potential receptors,
   - land use and human activities that could lead to exposure, and
   - receptor characteristics.

Typically in QRA, these are integrated into an estimate of exposure, e.g., in terms of potential human dose rate or concentration at the point of exposure to organisms. These types of measures are discussed further in the section titled "Structure for assessing exposure in CRS."

Davis et al. (1994) identified 34 different measures used for characterizing exposure in existing CRS systems. Examples of the use of these various measures and types of approaches for exposure include the following:

- The Wet Milieugevaarlijke Stoffen (WMS) Scoring System (Könemann and Visser 1988; Timmer et al. 1988) assigns scores for environmental exposure according to use volume, percentage released to the environment, degradation in air, soil, and/ or water, relative occurrence in these media, and bioconcentration. This system also scores exposure via products, including use patterns, exposure frequency, and intensity of exposure.

- The George Washington University (GWU) System (Foran and Glenn 1993) assesses exposure according to bioaccumulation, persistence, and release or production volume.

- The Effluent Monitoring Priority Pollutants List (EMPPL) (Environment Ontario 1987, 1988) includes environmental persistence, bioaccumulation, and detection in the environment.

- The German Beratergremium für Umweltrelevante Altstoffe (BUA) System (Behret 1989a, 1989b) includes bioaccumulation, persistence, and production volume.

- The USEPA Toxics Release Inventory (TRI) Environmental Indicators Methodology (Bouwes and Hassur 1997) uses facility-specific data and generic fate, transport, and exposure models to estimate a "surrogate dose," or the amount of chemical to which an individual might be exposed. The method includes a separate evaluation for each release pathway, allowing comparisons across media. The exposure scoring also includes the level of uncertainty. Exposure of aquatic life is obtained by estimates of the ambient water concentration.

- The Chemical Hazard Evaluation for Management Strategies (CHEMS-1) Model (Swanson et al. 1997) uses pounds of chemical released per year as reported in the TRI as a surrogate measure for potential exposure to human and environmental receptors.

- The Accelerated Reduction/Elimination of Toxics (ARET) Substance Selection Process (Environment Canada and OMOEE 1994) evaluates chemical bioaccumulation and persistence with environmental half-life ($t_{1/2}$), bioconcentration factor (BCF), and octanol–water partitioning coefficient (Kow) data.

- The Existing Chemicals System (Gjøs et al. 1989) uses chemical production and import volumes.

- The Pre-biologic Screen (Gillett 1983) uses Kow, Henry's Law constant (Hc), and $t_{1/2}$ to estimate bioaccumulation, persistence, and pervasiveness.

Further examples of systems using specific types of exposure measures are presented in the following section.

Characterizing Exposure in CRS

As exemplified by the approaches for characterizing exposure in existing CRS systems, a variety of measures may be applied separately or may be combined. These measures focus on chemical use and release, chemical properties and behavior, potential exposure-point concentrations, or on the exposure setting and possible human or ecological receptors. These types of exposure measures are used either explicitly in CRS or are used as the basis for scoring and ranking chemicals in some related way, as discussed below.

Using chemical marketing data

A variety of chemical marketing data sources have been used in existing CRS systems (based on Behret 1989a, 1989b; Walker and Brink 1989; Davis et al. 1994; Walker 1995). These include

- production volume or annual production volumes,
- import volume or annual import volumes,
- use volume,
- use pattern of the chemical, and
- number of sites of discharge or use.

Information such as chemical production and import volumes has been used as an indirect indicator of exposure to both humans and the environment. Gathering marketing data could be a very time-consuming process because there are many sources for these data. These data are available to regulators, although typically as confidential business information, e.g., as required by the U.S. Toxic Substances Control Act (TSCA) Inventory Update rule.

Examples of CRS systems that use marketing data include these:

- The Criteria to Identify Chemical Candidates for Sunsetting in the Great Lakes Basin system (Foran and Glenn 1993) uses annual chemical production and use volumes as criteria for evaluating chemicals manufactured, used, or stored in the Great Lakes Basin.
- The Systematic Data Collection and Handling for Priority Setting system (Gjøs et al. 1989) includes chemical production and import volumes as criteria for evaluating existing chemicals.

Using emission data

Several types of emission estimates have been used in existing CRS systems (based on Behret 1989a, 1989b; Walker and Brink 1989; Davis et al. 1994; Walker 1995). These include

- TRI emissions data,
- emission source data,
- waste volume,
- release reduction potential,
- fraction of chemical released in production facility, and
- fraction of chemical released to the environment from production.

Emission/release estimates reports

A useful source of information for estimating chemical releases might be any of the USEPA's or other government agency's reporting lists. The appropriate databases to include in a CRS system would depend on the purpose and application of that system. For example, the Criteria for Identifying High Risk Pollutants (USEPA 1991) uses national emissions data as criteria for scoring exposure potential for air pollutants.

Several USEPA reporting rules require manufacturers and users of the selected chemicals to provide information on releases and wastes resulting from chemical use. Examples include the USEPA's TRI program, tracking of wastewater and drinking water levels of the 129 priority pollutants, and the USEPA Office of Solid Waste's (OSW) Biennial Reporting System (BRS). The BRS contains information on quantities of hazardous waste generated and managed, although information on the mass of chemicals contained in these wastes often is not available. Many states and local governments have their own reporting systems that cover chemicals not covered by USEPA (e.g., pesticide use data by county in California).

Emission estimating techniques

Several databases contain different estimating methods for assessing environmental releases, e.g., the National Emission Database and compilation of Air Pollutant Emission Factors, AP-42 (USEPA 1995a). They usually provide information in either "amount released per amount used," "amount released per amount of production," or the types of equipment involved. These ratios are specific to the chemicals and to the process, and an understanding of the process is required to use these ratios.

Permitting data

Other sources of release estimates could be made using permitting information such as National Pollutant Discharge Elimination System (NPDES) permits or air permits. The NPDES permits are required for facilities discharging waste to surface water. NPDES permits and air permits specify both the amount of waste and the frequency of the release permitted at the facility, although the actual releases either may exceed or fail to reach the permitted values.

The data sources discussed above are applicable only if the chemicals of interest are included in the database. To estimate releases for chemicals not on any of the reporting/permitting lists, surrogate chemicals from the list could be used, where the surrogate chemical has similar chemical properties with similar processing or use.

Using physical–chemical properties

Existing CRS systems use a variety of physical–chemical properties (based on Behret 1989a, 1989b; Walker and Brink 1989; Davis et al. 1994; Walker 1995), including these:

- molecular weight (MW);
- water solubility;
- vapor pressure (Pv);
- Hc;
- penetrability of chemical into human or animal skin;
- BCF or bioaccumulation factor (BAF);
- soil–water and organic carbon–water partitioning coefficients (Kd, Koc);
- Kow;
- leaching potential;
- initial partitioning (Mackay [1991] Level I);
- environmental transfer factors (e.g., soil to plants, feed to cow milk, water purification, deposition, velocity, atmospheric dispersion);
- environmental spread (i.e., widespread versus localized use or emission); and
- degree of mobility.

Several chemical properties are important in assessing exposure. These properties indicate chemical behavior in the environment, particularly chemical movement from one medium to another or from one location to another. Typically, the transport properties of organic compounds easily may be evaluated in a systematic and semiquantitative way. It is somewhat more difficult to evaluate the behavior of inorganic chemicals released to the environment (e.g., metals, anions, mineral acids, and gases) where different approaches are required.

Inorganic chemicals

The transport of metals is highly site-specific and depends on soil pH, specification, sulfide/iron/magnesium concentration, presence of other metals and carbonates, ion exchange capacity, availability of oxygen, complexation, valence state, soil–water partition coefficient, and water solubility. Because of this strong dependence on site-specific information, the fate and transport of metals are difficult to characterize, especially for ranking and scoring purposes.

The transport behavior of anions is also highly site-specific. In general, anions are repelled by the negatively charged sites in the soil and tend not to remain sorbed to soil. For CRS, a simplifying assumption could be made that anionic chemicals reside exclusively in the aquatic compartment (i.e., in groundwater and surface water).

Characterizing the transport behavior of mineral acids may be simplified by assuming negligible sorption to most soils. Mineral acids released to the environment could therefore be assumed to ultimately reside in the aquatic compartment (groundwater and surface water).

The transport behavior of gases released to the environment may be simplified by assuming that gases will reside primarily in the air compartment. Water solubility of gases could also be considered.

Organic compounds

Although there are many physical properties reported for organic chemicals, a limited list of parameters should be sufficient for ranking purposes and environmental transport considerations. The following list of parameters represents the recommended set for organic compounds for CRS.

- Molecular weight is useful in assessing the transport of chemicals in the environment. Chemicals with lower MW tend to be more volatile, and chemicals with a higher MW are generally less soluble in water. The larger the MW, in general, the greater the tendency for sorption. Molecular weight also gives a general indication of molecular size, which affects uptake by fish; large molecules are not likely to bioconcentrate significantly.
- Water solubility indicates chemical tendency to leach to groundwater from the soil surface or vadose zone or to undergo transport in a subsurface aquifer. Water soluble and non-readily degradable compounds may be potential candidates for

groundwater contamination, plant uptake, and distribution in surface waters by dilution. The higher the water solubility, in general, the lower the tendency for sorption. Chemicals with high water solubility generally have less tendency to bioaccumulate in humans or other organisms.

- Vapor pressure indicates the tendency of a chemical to volatilize or evaporate. For chemicals dissolved in water or on moist soil, Hc is a better indicator of volatility. Pv is also important in determining whether a chemical in the atmosphere is present in the vapor phase or is partially or totally adsorbed to particulate matter.

- Henry's Law constant is a measure of chemical partitioning between air and water and indicates the potential for a chemical to volatilize from water or moist soil. Pervasiveness may be indicated by (dimensionless) log Hc > -4 (Gillett 1983).

- Dissociation constant (pKa) indicates the ionized and unionized forms of a chemical that exist in aqueous solution at varying pH and is important for ionizable chemicals such as acids or bases. Chemicals that ionize to an anionic form are less able to sorb to soils that contain negatively charged sites. Chemicals with low pKa tend to sorb weakly to soils and sediments and may be more mobile in the environment. Chemicals that form cations (e.g., amine) tend to sorb strongly to negatively charged clay material in soil.

- Bioconcentration factor is the ratio, at equilibrium, of chemical concentration in an exposed organism to the chemical concentration in the surrounding water. It is a measure of a chemical's tendency to bioaccumulate in fish or other organisms, and BCF can be measured experimentally or estimated from other properties such as Kow by QSAR. The BCF increases with increasing Kow until log Kow reaches approximately 6 (Bintein et al. 1993). Existing systems that consider BCF typically assign minimum scores (least concern) for log BCF values < 1 to < 2, and maximum scores (most concern) for log BCF > 3 to > 5, with moderate scores in between (Davis et al. 1994).

- Kow is a measure of a chemical's hydrophobicity and may be an important indicator of a chemical's tendency to partition between water in the environment and biota. Kow is often used to estimate BCF or other biota uptake factors.

- Koc gives a measure of a chemical's tendency to sorb to soil or sediment organic matter versus dissolving in water. An important indicator of leaching potential and groundwater transport, Koc is also important, along with Hc, in characterizing the potential for a chemical to volatilize from soil (e.g., Jury et al. 1983).

More information on these parameters is available in the literature (e.g., Howard 1989, 1990, 1991, 1992; Lyman et al. 1990).

Other parameters that may be useful include melting point, boiling point (BP), density, UV absorbance, evaporation rate, air diffusion coefficient, water diffusion coefficient, dermal penetrability, and environmental transfer factors (e.g., soil to plants, feed to cow milk). Information on the source of the data, and on the recommended methods when data are not available, is presented in the section titled "Data Issues."

CRS systems that use physical–chemical properties to characterize exposure

Chemical properties, especially BCF and Kow, are commonly used, alone or in combination with other measures, in existing CRS systems. For example, the Substances and Preparations Dangerous for the Environment system (Gustafsson and Ljung 1990) uses BCF or Kow; A Classification System for Hazardous Chemical Wastes (Crutcher and Parker 1990) uses Kd; and the Systematic Data Collection and Handling for Priority Setting system (Gjøs et al. 1989) includes log Kow, water solubility, and MW.

Using persistence and transformation processes

Chemical properties relating to persistence and transformation that have been used in CRS systems include the following (based on Behret 1989a, 1989b; Walker and Brink 1989; Davis et al. 1994; Walker 1995):

- degradability in air, water, soil and/or sediment (e.g., $t_{1/2}$);
- oxidation, photolysis, and/or hydrolysis rates;
- ratio of 5-day biological oxygen demand to chemical oxygen demand (BOD_5/COD);
- ratio of BOD_5 to theoretical oxygen demand (BOD_5 / THOD);
- qualitative degree of persistence, expert judgment;
- length of time contaminant source has been in existence (years);
- BOD half-life; and
- hydrolysis half-life.

These measures attempt to characterize several types of chemical degradation and transformation processes that may occur following release to the environment, either in air, water, or soil. These processes are discussed below.

Atmospheric photo-oxidation

Vapor-phase chemicals in the atmosphere (chemicals with Pv > ~ 10^{-4} torr) degrade mostly by photochemically generated hydroxyl radicals. With Pv below 10^{-4} torr, sorption to particulate matter becomes important, and atmospheric degradation is more difficult to determine. For a few chemicals, atmospheric reaction with ozone (e.g., olefinic and acetylenic chemicals) and nitrate radicals (e.g., phenols) is important.

Photolysis

Chemicals in air, in surface waters, and on soil surfaces can degrade by direct or indirect photochemical processes. For direct photolysis to be significant, a chemical must absorb sunlight (wavelengths in the ultraviolet spectrum greater than 290 nm), and the absorption of this energy must result in alteration of the chemical's structure. However, to be sure that a chemical directly photolyzes, experimental results are necessary, and only a few chemicals have appropriate experimental data. Methods for predicting direct photolysis are very limited (the only one proposed so far is for haloaromatic chemicals). Use of photolysis data in CRS is, therefore, very limited.

Sunlight can also generate oxidants such as alkoxy radicals in surface waters, especially waters with high humic content. These oxidants are found at high enough concentrations in surface waters that they will react at significant rates with some chemicals, e.g., phenols and furans, resulting in indirect photolysis.

Hydrolysis

Some chemicals have functional groups that are susceptible to abiotic hydrolysis under environmental conditions (e.g., carboxylic esters, carbamates, phosphate ester, haloalkanes). For these chemicals, hydrolysis may be important in soils and water. This process is usually pH- and temperature dependent. Hydrolysis half-life, estimated by QSAR, has been used as a measure of chemical persistence in water (Swanson et al. 1997).

Aerobic biodegradation

Aerobic biodegradation is a major factor in chemical persistence in soil and water and has considerable impact on the amount of chemical removal in most wastewater treatment plants. No known existing CRS systems have attempted to consider degradation products, and available data are limited. Most chemicals that biodegrade convert to more polar and oxidized chemicals that tend to biodegrade further. In contrast, photolysis and hydrolysis processes usually alter the chemical only slightly (e.g., photodieldrin) and only hydrolysis products can be predicted easily. Biological oxygen demand half-life, estimated by QSAR, also has been used as a measure of chemical persistence in water (Swanson et al. 1997).

Anaerobic biodegradation

Anaerobic ultimate biodegradation is a slower process than aerobic biodegradation, but may be important in certain settings (e.g., deep subsurface soil and groundwater). Anaerobic biodegradation data have not been used for ranking and scoring, probably because of the limited amount of data available in the past. For some chemicals, such as chlorinated hydrocarbons (transformed initially by dechlorination) and nitroaromatics (for which reduction of a nitro group to an amine is the first step), anaerobic biodegradation will be an important fate process that could be used to qualify a ranking or ordering of chemicals.

CRS systems that use chemical persistence or degradation properties

Examples of the use of qualitative measures of degradability in CRS include Existing Chemical of Environmental Relevance and the BUA Second Priority List (Behret 1989a,

1989b), which use qualitative indications of degradability or measured half-lives in air and water as 2 of their criteria in assessing chemicals.

Using monitoring data or other measured concentrations

A variety of monitoring data sources have been used in existing CRS systems (based on Behret 1989a, 1989b; Walker and Brink 1989; Davis et al. 1994; Walker 1995), including these:

- frequency of occurrence or detection;
- frequency of application;
- occurrence in air, soil, and/or water;
- maximum detected concentration;
- measured concentrations;
- concentration of introduced chemical (effluent monitoring data);
- concentrations in animal tissue, fish tissue, human tissue;
- concentrations in drinking water, groundwater, surface water;
- concentrations in workplace air, rural air, urban air; and
- theoretical daily dose (as a concentration) from HazDat database measured site concentrations.

Identification of a chemical in environmental and biota samples is ordinarily a reliable indicator of the potential for exposure. Monitoring data are available for only a small number of chemicals that could be subject to scoring or ranking. Inconsistencies in analytical methods, detection limits, units, etc., from one survey to another make it difficult to obtain a consistent dataset for any group of chemicals.

Monitoring data usually appear in the literature as an average, a maximum, and/or a range of concentrations. Frequency of detection or occurrence is also reported in many studies. USEPA's (1992c) Inventory of Exposure-Related Data Systems Sponsored by Federal Agencies provides descriptions of databases and contacts for other sources of exposure data, with a focus on measured environmental concentrations.

Monitoring data can be classified by environmental compartments, e.g., air, water, soil, sediment, and biota. The compartments can be subclassified for air as ambient, workplace, and indoor air; for water as drinking, surface, and groundwater; and for biota as animal, human, food, invertebrates, and plants.

One example of a CRS system that uses site-specific, measured environmental concentrations is the concentration/toxicity screen, described in USEPA's Risk Assessment Guidance for Superfund (USEPA 1989b), where the highest measured concentrations at a site are divided by reference doses (RfDs) and/or multiplied by cancer slope factors to identify chemicals of potential concern for the site.

Using modeled or estimated concentrations

Estimated ambient concentrations in air, water, soil, sediment, and/or biota have been used in several CRS systems (Davis et al. 1994). Although concentrations can be esti-mated using simple fate and transport models, sophisticated, data-intensive modeling to more accurately estimate environmental concentrations should be reserved for the high-est tier of CRS. Data required to estimate chemical concentration typically include chemical properties, chemical degradation rates, environmental and/or site characteris-tics, and chemical release or emission rates.

The estimation of chemical environmental concentrations may involve the use of generic environmental models (e.g., Mackay-type multi-media models). The standardized envi-ronmental parameters can be combined with emission rates and chemical fate data to estimate environmental concentrations in specific environmental media. Cowan et al. (1995) describe the use of multi-media fate models for predicting the fate of chemicals and the application of these models to environmental decision-making.

There are several different levels of these multi-media models. The Mackay Level I and II models are quite suitable to lower- and middle-tier CRS because they require the input of physical–chemical data that are often readily available, such as ambient temperature, MW, water solubility, Pv, and Hc. The more sophisticated Mackay Level III model (Mackay 1991) is a 4-compartment, steady-state model, which takes into account chemi-cal transport, advective flow, and degradation rates to estimate concentrations, percent distribution, compartment residence times, and intermediate transfer rates for air, water, soil, and sediment compartments. The Level III model is best suited for upper tier CRS because it requires considerably more data than the Level I and II models, and for many substances, the environmental behavior data needed are either unavailable or not readily available. All of the Mackay models mentioned above use a standardized "unit world" where the volumes of each compartment are defined. They are primarily designed for modeling the behavior of organic compounds, which can more easily be generalized than that of metals or other inorganic species.

The Uniform System for the Evaluation of Substances (Vermeire et al. 1994) uses a Mackay Level III-type model to evaluate regional environmental distributions of chemi-cals. Other CRS systems have been developed that use multi-media fate and transport modeling in some manner to evaluate the exposure potential for receptors of interest. Four systems documented by Davis et al. (1994) use Mackay Level I modeling:

- The Environmental Hazard Ranking System (Klein et al. 1988) models chemical quantity in environmental compartments.
- The WMS Scoring System (Könemann and Visser 1988) estimates the relative occurrence of chemicals in air, soil, and water.
- The European Commission (EC) Proposal for Priority Setting of Existing Chemi-cal Substances (van der Zandt and van Leeuwen 1992) uses Mackay Level I mod-eling to evaluate aquatic exposure.

- The Ontario MOE Scoring System (OMOE 1990) uses Mackay Level I modeling as part of its "multimedia partitioning" parameter to predict the number of environmental media a contaminant is likely to enter.

Another example of modeling concentrations is the Criteria for Identifying High Risk Pollutants (USEPA 1991), which estimates ambient air concentrations using USEPA's Human Exposure Model as a criterion for scoring exposure potential for air pollutants.

Alternatives to estimating concentrations include

- estimating chemical fraction in air, water, soil, sediment, and biota using chemical fate properties and partitioning models and
- estimating relative persistence in various media using chemical fate properties, partitioning models, and standard media residence times (See Example 2-2 at the end of this chapter).

Using receptor characteristics and exposure setting

A number of receptor or other exposure characteristics have been used in existing CRS systems (based on Behret 1989a, 1989b; Walker and Brink 1989; Davis et al. 1994; Walker 1995). These include (using the systems' terminology)

- number of workers exposed to chemical,
- consumer exposure,
- number of people in general population exposed to chemical,
- frequency of general population exposure to chemical,
- frequency of exposure,
- intensity of general population exposure to chemical,
- intensity of exposure,
- length of exposure,
- probability of exposure,
- plurality of exposure, and
- geographical extent of exposure (ecological).

Chemical ranking and scoring can be applied to a specific setting, i.e., a specific facility, site, or product, or it can be applied more generically. Both specific and generic approaches are discussed in the section titled "Structure for Assessing Exposure in CRS."

Release of chemicals to land, air, or water (the ambient environment) may result in exposure of both human and nonhuman populations. Monitoring data offer a measure of potential exposure at the time samples are collected, but data are available for only a small fraction of the universe of chemicals. The potential for ambient exposure is often estimated using data on chemical release amounts or release rates and knowledge of the chemical's environmental fate.

Non-ambient exposure includes consumer and occupational (indoor) settings. A large population may be exposed to a chemical if it is used directly by consumers or is present in a consumer product. The possibility of consumer exposure can itself be used as a simple input parameter in CRS. Exposure can be estimated with information on the consumer product and the concentration and total volume of the chemical used in that product.

Worker exposures can be measured or estimated. Several efforts in the industrial hygiene community have explored the topic of estimating worker exposures. There are data on worker exposure for chemicals now in use, particularly those regulated under the Occupational Safety and Health Act. Many of the data result from internal business efforts to monitor worker exposure and thus are not widely available. Some data generated by National Institute for Occupational Safety and Health (NIOSH) or Occupational Safety and Health Administration (OSHA) studies may be available to the public.

One example is the National Occupational Exposure Survey (NOES) (NIOSH 1988, 1990). It contains data that can be used to estimate both the number of workers and the number of use sites for an individual chemical. The NOES survey was a nationwide data-gathering effort by the NIOSH conducted in 1981. The survey was done to estimate the number of workers potentially exposed to various chemical, physical, and biological agents and the distribution of those potential exposures. Another example is the Census of Manufacture survey done by the U.S. Department of Labor Bureau of Labor Statistics (US BLS 1995). The census data list estimated number of workers and sites by 4-digit standard industrial classification (SIC) code.

Characterization of worker exposures to pollutants in the workplace is quite complex because it involves the interaction of worker behaviors and variable concentrations of contaminants in the workplace. The concentration patterns often are not constant but depend strongly on the nature of the work activities. In estimating the dose rates and frequencies, detailed information on the process is required. An alternative to such modeling that is more appropriate for CRS is to assume compliance with the OSHA permissible exposure limit (PEL) if a PEL has been set for the chemical of interest.

Examples of CRS systems that use receptor information include the Chemical Use Clusters Scoring Methodology (USEPA 1993a), which considers consumer use, the number of potentially exposed workers, and the number of use sites in assessing potential human exposure. Also, "plurality of direct exposure" (personal, domestic, and professional exposure) and the size of the risk population are considered in A Practical Method for Priority Selections and Risk Assessments among Existing Chemicals (Sampaolo and Binetti 1989). The International Testing Committee (ITC) Chemical Scoring System considers the number of workers exposed, number of consumers exposed, number of people exposed in the general population, and the frequency and intensity of exposure (Walker 1995). The ITC exposure scoring factors and criteria are shown in Example 2-1.

Using exposure expressed as intake

A generic equation to estimate chemical intake is

$$I = (EPC)(CR)(EF)(ED) / [(BW)(AT)] \qquad (2\text{-}1)$$

where

I = intake or exposure expressed as a potential dose rate (mg/kg/d);

EPC = chemical exposure point concentration (average concentration contacted over the exposure period);

CR = contact rate (the amount of chemical-containing medium contacted per unit time or exposure event [e.g., mg^3/day of air inhaled, 1/day of water ingested]);

EF = exposure frequency (days/year);

ED = exposure duration (years);

BW = body weight (the average bodyweight over the exposure period); and

AT = averaging time (days) (the time period over which exposure is averaged).

Intake is a measure of exposure expressed as the mass of a substance in contact with one of the exchange boundaries of an organism (i.e., skin, gastrointestinal tract, or lungs) per unit body weight per unit time (e.g., mg/kg/d). In this context, the term "potential dose rate" is more accurate; the concepts of intake, uptake, and dose are described in detail in the USEPA's Guidelines for Exposure Assessment (1992a).

It should be noted that characterizing exposure as estimated intake to a human receptor approaches the level of analysis done for QRA. Although there are examples of CRS systems expressing exposure potential in these terms, this level of analysis is neither typical nor recommended for most CRS applications. The use of intake, coupled with assessment of health effects, represents the highest tier of CRS (and, some would assert, approaches QRA rather than CRS). Based on Davis et al. (1994), measures of estimated intake or dose used in existing CRS systems include human exposure potential (in mg/kg/d) and estimated daily dose.

Concentration estimates may be integrated across all media (e.g., air, water, soil, and biota) using representative intake rates as the weighting factors. This approach is reflected as

$$E \,(\text{mg/kg/d}) = [\,Ia * Ca + Iw * Cw + \dots\,] / BW \qquad (2\text{-}2)$$

where

Ix = typical contaminant intake rate from medium x,

Cx = estimated concentrations of contaminants medium x, and

BW = body weight.

There may be significant temporal and spatial variations in the concentrations of contaminants in the various media. There are also substantial variations from person to person and from day to day in intake rates from the various media. However, these variations are ignored here; the relevant concentrations are averaged over time and space, and the relevant intake rates are averaged over population and activity pattern. In this approach, variation is important only to the extent that it influences the average value of the parameter of interest.

Although there are spatial and temporal variations in air pollutant concentrations, if these are not correlated with variations in population density, the average rate of exposure can be estimated by multiplying the average intake and the average concentration. This principle also applies to the other pathways.

One CRS system that uses estimated dose is the TRI Environmental Indicators Methodology (Bouwes and Hassur 1997), which uses TRI release data, fate and transport modeling, and information about populations near TRI reporting facilities to estimate "human exposure potential" expressed as a dose rate (mg/kg/day). This is not typical, however, of most CRS systems.

Structure for Assessing Exposure in CRS

This section describes the use of exposure measures in various combinations or levels of sophistication. The usefulness of the CRS results is largely dependent on the timeliness, pertinence, and the degree of uncertainty inherent in the score.

Sequential analysis

Chemical ranking and scoring systems span a wide range of complexity. One theme that was stressed in this workshop was the need for tiered CRS analysis. The conceptual model for CRS (Figure 1-2) shows successive CRS tiers as the level of analysis of the components (ecological and health effects, exposure, other chemical characteristics) increases or becomes more sophisticated.

Much of the difference in complexity from one CRS system to another is due to the large variation in approaches for assessing exposure. For example, a CRS system using simple measures (such as chemical–physical properties) as surrogates for exposure would be much less sophisticated, and therefore a lower tier than one using exposure measures more closely approximating exposure point concentrations or even intakes.

Two aspects to levels of complexity in assessing exposure for CRS can be distinguished. One aspect is how specific the analysis is regarding the location or exposure setting. Chemicals can be assessed without any consideration for the setting, using standard assumptions about a typical setting, or can be assessed by focusing on a specific site, location, facility, or even on a specific manufactured product. This is represented in Figure 2-1 as a "generic" or "specific" setting.

		Generic setting	Specific setting
↑ Increasing level of sophistication ↑	**Potential dose rates**	Estimated dose rate (mg/kg/d): exposure point concentrations, standardized intake model assumptions	Estimated dose rate (mg/kg/d): exposure point concentrations, site-specific intake parameters
	Concentrations	Concentrations in various media: chemical fate properties, emission rates, media characteristics	Estimated concentrations: fate and transport models, site-specific parameters
		Relative persistence in various media: chemical fate properties, partitioning models, standard media residence times	Measured concentrations, monitoring data
		Chemical fraction in air, water, soil/sediment, biota: chemical fate properties, partitioning models	
	Surrogate measures	Chemical fate properties	Facility- or location-specific chemical emission data: e.g., TRI, NPDES
		Aggregated emission data	
		Aggregated PUD[1] data	Product PUD[1] data: e.g., LCA inventory data

[1] PUD = production, use, and disposal

Figure 2-1 Matrix of exposure tiers in CRS

The other aspect is how closely the exposure assessment or exposure measures approach those typically used in QRA. Ecological risk assessment typically uses estimated or measured chemical concentrations in the media of concern where organisms may come in contact (the point of exposure). For human health risk assessment, chemical concentrations at the exposure point are typically combined with intake models to estimate a potential dose rate, usually expressed as mg chemical per kg body weight per day. Exposure levels in various media, expressed as concentrations, may also be used for human health assessments. (There are other, more accurate measures of exposure used in QRA, such as measured tissue levels, biomarkers, or biokinetic uptake models, but these are beyond the scope of this discussion.) At the other end of the spectrum, surrogate measures for exposure, such as annual emission data or chemical fate parameters are often used in CRS to quantify, in a simple way, some aspect of the potential for exposure to the chemical. This aspect of CRS structure is referred to in this discussion as the "degree of sophistication."

Resource requirements and the level of effort required to score chemicals increases with numbers of chemicals scored and with the level of sophistication employed in the method. The appropriate degree of sophistication depends on the uncertainty of the first tier and the potential consequences, i.e., the costs associated with decisions based on the CRS results.

Four of the boxes in Figure 2-1 are discussed below in more detail. Surrogate exposure measures can vary from generic to specific settings and are discussed in the sections titled "Generic exposure setting" and "Specific exposure setting." The working group could not reach agreement as to whether using concentrations is appropriate for CRS. This is also discussed in both the generic and specific setting sections. The upper 2 boxes, representing potential dose rates, were not considered generally appropriate for CRS and are not discussed further.

Different approaches to assessing exposure in CRS would be appropriate, depending on the purpose and application of the system as well as the time and resources available. The approach should also be consistent with the approach taken in assessing human health, ecological, and other impacts and with the overall framework of the system.

One important consideration in a tiered approach is the preservation of data from simpler to more sophisticated tiers. As the analysis moves up the scale from simple surrogate measures to more sophisticated estimates, the information used in the previous level should remain apparent and usable in later levels. As one moves up in the levels shown in Figure 2-1 for a generic setting, previous data are retained and combined with added information to make more sophisticated assessments. For instance, exposure potential in a generic setting could be scored using chemical fate parameters and national emission rates for a "tier a" analysis. Then the same fate parameters could be combined with assumptions about a standardized environment in a multimedia equilibrium partitioning model to estimate expected fractions in various environmental media, for a "tier b" analysis. Or the fate parameters and emission rates could be combined with degradation rates in a model to estimate environmental concentrations at steady state. If QRA were deemed necessary for some chemicals, the fate parameters, emission rates, degradation rates, and perhaps the estimated concentrations would all be useful information.

Another important aspect is the incorporation of feedback loops or triggers, to indicate when further evaluation of a chemical is warranted.

Generic exposure setting

Generic settings typically apply to nationally aggregated data or simply to unspecified locations.

Surrogate exposure measures

Surrogates are parameters that are more easily measured, or for which data are readily available, and that are expected to correlate with actual or potential exposure. They are commonly used as substitutes for more sophisticated estimates of exposure. Use of surrogate measures in a generic setting may include the following, alone or in some combination, to classify, score, or rank chemicals:

- nationally aggregated chemical marketing, or PUD data;
- nationally aggregated emission rates, such as the annual TRI data;
- chemical fate properties;
- chemical degradation rates; and
- number exposed or potentially exposed (workers, consumers, or general population).

Twenty-four of the fifty-one risk ranking systems examined by Davis et al. (1994) used chemical fate properties alone to evaluate exposure. Although the choice of fate properties might imply media of concern, the CRS analysis at this level does not focus on any specific location or process. Example 2-1 presents the exposure, persistence, bioaccumulation potential factors, and criteria developed by the ITC; these are used by USEPA's new and existing chemical programs and others to score and rank chemicals (Walker 1995).

Estimated or relative chemical concentrations

Three CRS systems examined by Davis et al. (1994) used estimated chemical concentrations in a generic setting to evaluate exposure. An approach that considers partitioning and persistence in environmental compartments, providing relative concentrations in various environmental media, is presented in Example 2-2.

Specific exposure setting

Chemical ranking and scoring is also applied to a specific known setting such as an industrial facility, a National Priority List (NPL) site, etc.

Surrogate exposure measures

The CRS process at the lower right-hand portion of Figure 2-1 is concerned with emission rates, uses, and site-specific characteristics of large numbers of chemicals and environments. Two CRS systems examined by Davis et al. (1994) use surrogate measures to evaluate exposure in a specific setting.

The Region VII Toxics Release Inventory Geographic Risk Analysis System (TRIGRAS) (Bouchard 1991) ranks risk to both human and ecological health from TRI releases for specified geographic areas. The system uses TRI release amounts (by county or zip code) and stream volumes to determine "relative daily toxic loadings" to specific areas.

The International Joint Commission's (IJC) Binational Objective Committee (1989) developed the Great Lakes Water Quality Agreement Annex Lists 1, 2, and 3, also using surrogate exposure measures for a specific location. Here, exposure potential was determined by whether a substance either was present in the Great Lakes or had the potential of being discharged to the Great Lakes in consideration of a suite of possible toxic effects.

Estimated or measured concentrations

For some sites, a list of detected chemicals needs to be narrowed down to select chemicals of concern for QRA. For hazardous waste site investigations, measured concentrations are available or concentrations have been estimated using fate and transport modeling. Although not the most common application, this is a case where CRS may be appropriate.

Six CRS systems examined by Davis et al. (1994) used estimated or measured chemical concentrations to evaluate exposure in a specific setting. For example, the new Pollutant Standards Index (USEPA 1978) used measured air pollutant concentrations at a specific location to calculate a daily index for public information about air quality.

Data Issues

Data issues discussed in this section include data sources and methods for estimating missing data, data quality, data availability, and uncertainty.

Data sources and estimating methods

Table 2-1 lists sources and estimating methods for chemical properties data. An additional discussion of data sources is provided in Appendix B, titled "Sources of Data for Chemical Ranking and Scoring Purposes." A detailed discussion of estimating methods and data quality is beyond the scope of this chapter; the reader is referred to the literature for more information (e.g., Howard 1989, 1990, 1991, 1992; Lyman 1990).

Uncertainties

Uncertainties in estimates of risk (Finkel 1990) arise due to the following:
- uncertainties related to the type of decision to be made, particularly categorical uses of the assessment (decision or scenario uncertainty);
- fundamental limitations in scientific understanding of the processes governing environmental fate and transport (process or model uncertainty);
- imprecision in estimates of key parameters of the model (parameter uncertainty); or
- stochastic variation in the data.

The issues of uncertainty and variability in risk assessment are addressed in detail elsewhere (e.g., USEPA 1992a). Regarding CRS, relevant issues include acknowledging and evaluating uncertainty and variability in a ranking method and how these may affect the decision-making process the CRS is to support.

Parameter uncertainty

One important consideration is that chemical properties are typically measured in a controlled laboratory setting. In laboratory tests, a pure compound is typically used, whereas the same chemical in the environment may interact with other substances, possibly influencing the chemical properties. The laboratory setting generally represents ideal behavior where the influence of other substances is minimal. Chemicals found in the environment may deviate from ideal conditions to a varying extent. Other potentially important uncertainties include the need to estimate parameter values and the variation within individual parameters due to different measuring and/or estimating methods.

One approach to addressing uncertainty would be to develop probabilistic frameworks for chemical scoring. Probabilistic characterization of chemical scores would have at least 2 potential benefits. Users would be less likely to misuse the scores, and analysts would be better able to decide whether a first tier analysis was adequate or whether more complex procedures were necessary.

Table 2-1 Sources of data for exposure measures

Parameter	Sources of data	Estimating methods
Molecular weight (MW)	Merck Index (Budavari et al. 1996) or obtained from the chemical structure.	MW may also be used to estimate a variety of other important physical properties (Lyman et al. 1990).
Water solubility	Commercial databases (e.g., Hazardous Substances Data Bank [HSDB] available from the National Library of Medicine; Yalkowsky et al. [1989]). Printed sources: Horvath 1982; USEPA 1986; Howard 1989, 1990, 1991, 1992; Shiu et al. 1990; Mackay et al. 1992.	May be estimated from log Kow with various available regression equations (Lyman et al. 1990; Meylan et al. 1996).
Octanol-water partition coefficient (Kow)	HSDB; USEPA 1986; Hansch and Leo 1987; Howard 1989, 1990, 1991, 1992; Mackay et al. 1992; Sangster database. 10,000+ chemicals have measured values.	Estimated from water solubilities (Lyman et al. 1990) or from chemical structure for almost any organic chemical with a mean error of approximately 0.30 log units (e.g., CLOGP from Biobyte, Inc. [1996] and LOG Kow [Meylan and Howard 1995]).
Organic carbon-water partition coefficient (Koc)	Experimental values of Koc and leaching studies are available in the Environmental Fate Data Base (EFDB; SRC 1994), in Howard et al. (1986), and in HSDB.	Estimated from water solubility or Kow (Lyman et al. 1990) or from structure (Meylan et al. 1992).
Vapor pressure (Pv)	HSDB, EFDB; Boublik et al. 1984; Riddick et al. 1986; USEPA 1986; Daubert and Danner 1989; Howard 1989, 1990, 1991, 1992; Mackay et al. 1992; Wauchope et al. 1992.	Programs such as PCCHEM from USEPA's OPPT or MPBPVP from Syracuse Research Corporation estimate Pv from an estimated boiling point that can be estimated from structure or use a measured value.
Henry's Law constant (Hc)	HSDB; Hine and Mookerjee 1975; Mackay and Shiu 1981; Shiu and Mackay 1986; USEPA 1986; Howard 1989, 1990, 1991, 1992; Mackay et al. 1992.	Estimated from Pv and water solubility (Lyman et al. 1990) or from structure (Meylan and Howard 1991).
Acid dissociation constant (pKa)	Perrin IUPAC report, etc.; EFDB (SRC 1994).	Estimated by various programs, most of which rely on linear free energy relationships (LFER).
Bioconcentration factor (BCF)	Experimental data are available from the USEPA AQUIRE database, EFDB (SRC 1994), and HSDB.	Estimated from Kow, S, MW (Veith et al. 1979; Briggs 1981; Lyman et al. 1990).
Hydrolysis rate	Mabey and Mill (1978) and reports (e.g., Ellington et al. 1987; EFDB [SRC 1994]) on a limited number of chemicals (several hundred).	Estimation methods for predicting rate constants are available but will apply only to certain classes of chemicals (e.g., Hamrick et al. 1992; Kollig 1993).
Anaerobic biodegradation rate	EFDB (SRC 1994) and HSDB; data are primarily available for pesticides, because there is a standard protocol (flooded soil) and data ordinarily are required for pesticide registration. Test data are available for only several hundred chemicals.	No estimating methods are available.

Table 2-1 *continued*

Parameter	Sources of data	Estimating methods
Aerobic biodegradation	The BIODEG file (Howard et al. 1987, about 700 chemicals) in EFDB (SRC 1994) and HSDB (about 1200 chemicals). The BIODEG file has summary codes that could be used in a ranking scheme; HSDB; biodegradation data on over 6,000 chemicals have been indexed in the BIOLOG file (Howard et al. 1986) of EFDB.	Methods for estimating from structure are available (e.g., Enslein et al. 1984; Neimi et al. 1986; Boethling et al. 1994; Klopman et al. 1995).
Photo-oxidation	Hydroxyl radical rate constants have been reviewed by Atkinson (1994) for approximately 400 chemicals, and these values have been used to calculate an atmospheric half-life by assuming an average hydroxyl radical rate constant.	Atkinson (1987) has also developed a method for estimating hydroxyl radical rate constants for most organic chemicals; a computer program is available for calculating estimated values from structure (Meylan and Howard 1993).
Photolysis rate	A few chemicals have direct and indirect photolysis data in EFDB (SRC 1994) and HSDB.	Endpoints cannot be estimated.
Chemical marketing information	U.S. International Trade Commission, trade journals, Kirk-Othmer, Chemical Buyers' Guide, Mannsville Chemical Products Synopsis.	Not applicable.
Monitoring data	HSDB; annual technical reports from USEPA, e.g., the National Human Adipose Tissue Survey (NHATS), U.S. Geological Survey, the Food and Drug Administration.	Not applicable.
Consumer use	Clinical Toxicology of Commercial Products searched by chemical constituent and product use, the HSDB Consumer Products Safety Commission's System for Tracking Inventory of Chemicals (includes codes indicating whether the chemical is found in a consumer product), USEPA's Indoor Air Chemical Source database.	Not applicable.

Scenario uncertainty

Scenario uncertainty is particularly difficult to address in CRS because it often requires different types of models to be applied to different portions of the data.

Human exposure assessments directed at occupational health or consumer product safety are markedly different from the general population exposure or the exposure to humans as a part of the ecosystem. The scientific techniques and modeling assumptions are disparate, and radically different concerns surface. For example, acute toxicity is more of a concern in occupational settings where exposure to higher concentrations is more likely than in the ambient environment (although chronic exposure may also be of concern). Therefore, segregating the scenarios for human non-environmental impact from the general environmental impact scenarios is recommended.

Model uncertainty

Model uncertainties arise from limitations in current understanding of the phenomena of interest. A common tendency is to characterize only the data and parameter uncertainties because this can be done objectively. This may be misleading because the most significant uncertainties in estimating risks are often due to model or scenario uncertainty.

Variability

In addressing uncertainty, it is helpful to make a distinction between variability and uncertainty. An uncertain quantity is one that has a (single) true, but unknown, value; a variable quantity is one that takes on different values over space, time, or among individuals. Whereas uncertainty can be reduced by research, variability is a fundamental characteristic of the processes of interest. Although the degree of variability may be uncertain, and therefore a subject for research itself, research will not reduce the underlying true variability in the system. Probability distributions are typically used to characterize uncertain quantities, and frequency distributions are used to characterize variable quantities.

No simple scoring or ranking procedure can involve complex dynamic modeling of the exposures of workers, consumers, or those living near production facilities. However, in principle, it would be possible to characterize the stochastic variability in emissions, transport, and dispersion processes and to integrate across these to obtain simple indices of exposure that could account for these effects. Unfortunately, currently the data and analyses needed for this approach are not readily available.

Findings and Recommendations

General findings of the Exposure Assessment Workgroup are, first, that assessing exposure for CRS is a complex issue and that many approaches to assessing potential exposure have been developed and used in existing CRS systems. Second, guidance exists for exposure assessment in quantitative risk assessment, but that level of detail typically is not appropriate for CRS.

Recommended principles for assessing exposure in CRS include the following:
- Uncertainty should be described along with the results.
- The degree of sophistication should be appropriate to the decision-making.

- An iterative approach should be used with feedback loops built in, starting at simplest level.
- Data should be preserved, as much as possible, from one level to the next.

Summary and Recommendations for Future Work

This chapter discussed measures of exposure for CRS, specifically types of measures used for exposure, parameters, data sources, structure of levels or tiers, and uncertainties. Recommendations for future work include these:

- Integrate exposure with human health, ecological, and other chemical characteristics into an overall CRS framework.
- Further develop suggested approaches and applications for the different tiers of exposure assessment.
- Further develop appropriate methods to estimate missing data.
- Validate or verify scoring methods.
- Integrate often-used environmental fate and exposure data into databases suitable for CRS purposes. A specific example of this would be anaerobic biodegradation data, perhaps building upon the SRC/USEPA BIODEG file (Howard et al. 1986).

Example 2-1: ITC exposure factors, scores, and criteria

Exposure factors	Scores and criteria for assigning exposure scores			
	3	2	1	0
Annual production volume (millions of pounds)	≥ 100	≥ 10	≥ 1	≤ 1
Fraction released to the environment (percent)	> 30	3 to 30	0.3 to 3	< 0.3
Number of workers exposed (in thousands)	≥ 100	≥ 10	≥ 1	≤ 1
Number of consumers exposed (in thousands)	≥ 10	≥ 1	≥ 0.1	≤ 0.1
Number of people exposed in general population (in millions)	> 20	2 to 20	0.2 to 2	< 0.2
Frequency of exposure	Daily	Weekly	Monthly	Yearly
Intensity of exposure	High (solvents)	Medium (dust)	Low (dyes)	Very low (intermediates)
Penetrability of chemical into human or animal skin (percent) [1]	10 to 100	1 to 10	0.01 to 1	< 0.01
Persistence of chemical in the environment	Years	Months	Days	Hours
Bioaccumulation potential (Log Kow)	> 5	3 to 5	1 to 3	< 1

[1] Walker et al. (1996) provide data for skin penetrability. Other potential data sources are listed in Table 3-1.
Source: Walker 1995.

Example 2-2: Partitioning and Persistence in Environmental Compartments

The use of generic exposure setting to evaluate the potential for chemical exposure to atmospheric, terrestrial, benthic, and aquatic compartments is discussed below. Screening can be performed from fate parameters regarding persistence, pervasiveness, and bioaccumulation potential.

Steps include these:

- Apportion released chemical between water, soil, and air (initial partitioning).
- Indicate the extent or role of persistence, either for a unit time or for a surrogate of media retention time.
- Modify initial partitioning using degradation factor (DF).
- Estimate further partitioning into biota.

Based on this screen, chemicals can be identified as 1) persistent in biota or soil/sediment or 2) as mobilized to air or groundwater.

The system requires the following inputs (Figure 2-2 presents an overview):

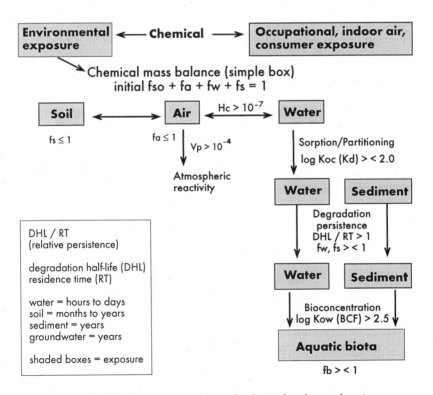

Figure 2-2 Generic exposure assessment for chemical ranking and scoring

- Hc or log Pv and S as a surrogate;
- sorption or partition coefficient, Koc (or Kd);
- Kow or BCF;
- $t_{1/2}$ in various environmental compartments (e.g., air, soil, water, sediment) or first order degradation rate (kb) (preferably as biodegradation, but photolysis and hydrolysis may be more important for certain structures); and
- estimated residence times for those environmental compartments.

STEP 1: initial partitioning

The fractional amount of chemical can be estimated in various media using Hc, Koc, and Kow, which can be experimentally measured values or QSAR estimates (see Table 2-1 for data sources).

First, determine the fraction of chemical in air (fa) based on Hc (the following criteria are suggested):
- Chemicals with Hc > 10^{-3} are extensively volatilized under almost all conditions and will partition almost exclusively into the atmospheric compartments (i.e., fa = 1).
- Chemicals that have Hc values between 10^{-6} and 10^{-4} will volatilize to various extents depending on environmental conditions (i.e., 0 < fa < 1).
- Volatility is estimated using a cutoff value for Hc of 10^{-7} atm/m^3/mole; chemicals that have a value less than 10^{-7} are considered nonvolatile (i.e., fa = 0).

Chemicals that are largely nonvolatile have the potential to sorb or partition to soil, sediment, and water compartments based on their partition (Koc) or sorption (Kd) coefficients. For chemicals with fa < 1, based on chemical mass balance, the fraction of chemical in soil–sediment or water compartments, plus the fraction of chemical in air, will be equal to 1:

$$fa + fso + fs + fw = 1 \qquad\qquad (2\text{-}3)$$

where

$$
\begin{aligned}
fa &= \text{fraction of chemical in air,} \\
fso &= \text{fraction of chemical in soil,} \\
fs &= \text{fraction of chemical in sediment, and} \\
fw &= \text{fraction of chemical in water.}
\end{aligned}
$$

Determining fa, fso, fs, and fw is outlined in Figure 2-2.

Relative fractions in water versus soil/sediment can be determined by Koc or Kd.

If log Kd or log Kow > 2, the chemical will primarily be adsorbed to soil or sediment.

STEP 2: Determine degradation half-life to residence time ratio and DF.

Two factors must be considered to estimate the potential for removal or accumulation in the environment:

- The rate of degradation or degradation half-life (DHL) in a particular environmental compartment. Extensive data on the chemical and biological degradation of a variety of chemicals have shown that degradation kinetics can be described by a first-order reaction. (First-order degradation means that the rate of degradation is directly proportional to chemical concentration and largely independent of other environmental variables.) Because the rate of degradation varies directly with the concentration of the chemical during first-order degradation, the DHL is most often used to compare the degradation kinetics of chemicals. The DHL is derived from the first -order degradation rate constant and is independent of the chemical concentration. It is operationally defined as the time required to reduce the concentration of the chemical to 50% of its original value, or to yield half the maximal amount of the end-product, and is calculated from the relationship $t_{1/2} = \ln 2/k_1$ $0.693/k$, where k_1 is the first-order degradation rate constant.

- The residence time (RT) of a chemical in that compartment. Typical residence times that might be used include 34 hours for surface water, 15 years for sediment, and 1 year for soil (Larson and Cowan 1995).

Chemicals are subject to degradation by biological or chemical mechanisms. Residence time represents the time available for degradation to occur. The importance of degradation is defined by the degradation half-life to residence time (DHL:RT) ratio. For a given environmental compartment, the potential for degradation or accumulation and persistence of a chemical can be characterized by DHL / RT.

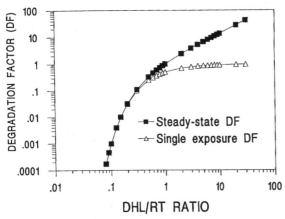

Figure 2-3 *Degradation factor versus DHL:RT ratio*

Potential degradation or accumulation can be quantified using degradation factors (DFs), where DF is determined from DHL / RT based on the relationship shown in Figure 2-3 (Larson and Cowan 1995). The degradation factor indicates the relative change in environmental exposure levels at a constant input rate and can be calculated for single or multiple (i.e., steady-state) exposures (see Figure 2-3).

When DHL is equal to RT (i.e., DHL / RT = 1), the following occur:
- The maximum mass loading of the chemical in the environment at steady state will approach, but not exceed, the input rate after biodegradation has occurred.
- The maximum concentration immediately after input will be twice the input rate (i.e., DF = 2) and will decrease over the course of the RT to approximate the steady-state value.
- Significant removal due to degradation (i.e., 50%) occurs in single-exposure situations when the DHL:RT ratio = 1.

When DHL is less than RT (i.e., DHL / RT < 1), the following occur:
- Between 0.2 and 0.3, the steady-state concentration will increase above the input rate. At DHL:RT ratios < 0.3, the steady-state concentration is less than 10% of the input rate and does not represent a significant fraction of the total amount of chemical present.
- At a DHL:RT ratio of 0.1 or less, however, degradation results in essentially complete removal of the chemical, and no detectable increases will occur. At smaller DHL:RT ratios, no significant accumulation above the input rate will occur (even immediately after input of the chemical); both single-exposure and steady-state concentrations will be comparable.

When DHL exceeds RT (i.e., DHL / RT > 1), the following occur:
- The chemical will accumulate in that compartment under steady-state conditions.
- At DHL:RT ratios of approximately 5 or greater, less than 15% removal will occur due to degradation.
- At high DHL:RT ratios, this accumulation can result in environmental concentrations that are orders of magnitude higher than the input loading rate. These high levels will persist for extended periods after the input has ceased, resulting in chemical concentrations that are orders of magnitude higher than those predicted on input rates alone.

STEP 3: Combine DF and initial fractions to obtain a (unitless) chemical score for each medium. Degradation factor values can be used to adjust the fraction of chemical remaining in sediment or water compartments, where

$$(DF_x)(f_x) = f_x', \text{ adjusted fraction of chemical in compartment } x.$$

The DF will be less than 1 if degradation is a practical removal mechanism and greater than 1 if accumulation is occurring. The fractional values for f_s and f_w, therefore, can also be adjusted to values less than or greater than 1, depending on the DF.

STEP 4: Further refine aquatic partitioning (with fw and bioconcentration)

Once persistence is refined (fw' is determined) in aquatic compartments, the potential for bioconcentration can be estimated from Kow or BCF. Fractional values for chemicals in the biotic compartment (fb) can be estimated by fw' and Kow or BCF. Significant uptake for biota is expected for log Kow (or log BCF) > 2.5. Values for fb will also be less than or greater than 1, depending on whether degradation or accumulation has increased or decreased fw.

The chemical fraction in sediment can be further evaluated to estimate the potential for benthic exposures. The relative changes in fw, fs, and fb from their initial values indicate the potential for degradation, persistence, and bioaccumulation of a chemical in aquatic and benthic compartments.

Chapter 3

Human Health Effects

Gary K. Hurlburt, chapter editor
Rolf Bretz, Emma Lou George, Rolf Hartung, Raymond Kent,
Lynne Fahey McGrath, Ron Newhook, Mike Stevens, Bradford Strohm, Pauline Wagner

The Human Health Effects Workgroup discussed the state of the science for chemical ranking and scoring (CRS) in general, then specifically as related to human health effects. The workgroup concluded that because there are numerous purposes for CRS, it would be impossible to create or recommend one specific system that would fit all potential uses. However, the workgroup did conclude that there were guiding principles by which all scoring and ranking systems would benefit:

- Common categories and subcategories that are important to multiple-purpose systems should be used.
- Inputs and decision-making processes should be simple to use.
- Category endpoints should be transferable directly to more complicated risk assessment activities, unencumbered as much as possible by value judgments or safety factors.
- Outputs should contribute to relative ranking but be value-neutral as to risk or safety.

Specifically, the workgroup considered the categories of acute toxicity, subchronic/chronic toxicity, and carcinogenicity to be generally important to CRS systems designed to evaluate adverse impacts to humans. The endpoints of no-observed-adverse-effect levels (NOAELs) and lowest-observed-adverse-effect levels (LOAELs) for threshold effects, and the effective dose for response in 10% of the population observed (ED10) from cancer potency models were considered value-neutral, comparable measures for relative ranking, which are transferable directly to the risk/safety assessment process. It was agreed that animal data may be used where human epidemiologic data are not available and that structure-activity relationship (SAR) estimations may be used for some applications where data are lacking.

The workgroup found it necessary and beneficial to visualize their deliberations via use of a very basic ranking and scoring paradigm. The paradigm summarizes the workgroup's conclusions that, although exposure assessment is not a necessary part of the health effects review, it defines the purpose for the review (i.e., the population, route, duration of potential exposure, etc.) and therefore must be considered in the final product. Further, modifiers that identify strengths and weaknesses in data and severity of endpoints must be addressed transparently and also factored into the relative ranking process. Although the workgroup did not attempt to develop the ideal ranking and scoring system, the paradigm used to visualize the process represents the general approach the workgroup would follow in developing a chemical ranking for human health effects. This includes knowing the specific purpose for the ranking and its application before designing the details of its inputs (i.e., categories, subcategories, exposures, modifying values, etc.).

State of the Science

Hundreds of CRS systems have been developed throughout the world. The University of Tennessee Center for Clean Products reviewed approximately 50 ranking and scoring systems and identified at least 68 endpoints being used to evaluate human health effects (Davis et al. 1994). These endpoints are measured, aggregated, weighted, scored, and/or ranked in a variety of different ways. Categories of effects considered may range from single-exposure acute effects to long-term exposure chronic effects. The type of effects considered may range from simple skin irritation to tumor development. The severity of effects may be as mild and reversible as enzyme induction or as irreversible and severe as lethality. Some systems are easy to use, requiring little sophistication and data, while others are quite complicated and data-intensive and require considerable knowledge in evaluating effects. Data use may range from estimations of potential effects derived from SARs to human epidemiological data. Weighting and ranking of effects in these systems range from the assignment of arbitrary numeric values or narrative descriptions for various dose-related effects, to more risk assessment-related endpoints of reference doses (RfDs), reference concentrations (RfCs), and cancer risk values (potency slope). Uses of these systems have ranged from simple screening of chemicals or categorizing chemicals by effect to complicated numeric hazard rankings for risk assessments.

Characterizing Human Health Effects

Three general categories for evaluating human health effects may be defined for use in a wide range of CRS applications: 1) acute toxicity, 2) subchronic/chronic toxicity, and 3) carcinogenicity. To avoid the arbitrary nature of numerical scores superimposed over adverse effects data, or potentially value-laden "uncertainty" factors applied, it is suggested that the most sensitive effect/no-effect levels should be used in relative ranking. Davis et al. (1994) have identified at least 9 CRS systems that currently use either no-observed-effect level (NOEL), NOAEL, or LOAEL as a decision endpoint.

In many existing CRS systems, arbitrary cancer scores or model-dependent cancer potency slopes have an overpowering influence on scoring outcomes compared with the influence of noncancer effects. To relate cancer and noncancer effects on a more comparable basis, the use of an ED10 in mg/kg/d established from the cancer bioassay data, is preferred as a relative ranking value. Davis et al. (1994) have identified at least 5 scoring systems that currently use either the ED10 or some derivative thereof. However, the ED10 value for many carcinogens may not always be readily available, requiring the use of a weight-of-evidence classification evaluation for many ranking exercises. The ED10 may be then limited to a "modifier" role in differentiating between smaller groups of chemicals where the resources necessary to determine ED10 values are more limited. When ED10 values become more widely available in the literature, these values should be used preferentially with weight-of-evidence classification as a modifying factor. The United States Environmental Protection Agency's (USEPA 1996) Proposed Guidelines for Carcinogen Risk Assessment recommends the use of an ED10; therefore, the estimation of ED10 values for cancer endpoints may become more common and their use in CRS more widely applicable.

The effect level measured for these 3 major categories may be subject to further evaluation to take into account such factors as severity of effect, potency, data quality and quantity, and other endpoints such as mutagenicity. Many current scoring systems include mutagenicity as a major component. However, mutagenicity data may not be directly applicable to an uncomplicated scoring system due to lack of comparability (on a mg/kg/d basis) with the categories of acute toxicity, subchronic/chronic toxicity, and carcinogenicity. Evidence of mutagenicity may be important as a modifier in the relative ranking of a chemical, but considerable expertise is required to interpret the relevance of such data to human health concerns, which may preclude their use in some CRS applications. Best professional judgment should be applied on a case-by-case basis in developing modifiers that address other factors not discussed here.

The appraisal of effects of chemicals on human health is best done using epidemiological data, but often these data are lacking or are limited with respect to exposure information and the details of the description of the effects. Consequently, it is often necessary to use data derived from studies on laboratory animals. These encompass a broad span of exposure conditions and effects, e.g., exposure durations ranging from acute through subchronic to chronic and effects ranging from the obvious (such as death) to the subtle. It should be recognized that some animal species and strains have unique physiological or biochemical characteristics different from those of humans, which may bring into question their relevance as human models.

Effects due to short-term exposures

Acute effects

In general, acute toxicity data should be included in the health effects assessment of a CRS system. It represents the largest and most widespread source of toxicological information for ranking and scoring systems. Also, there is a long tradition of using these data to categorize and label chemicals and to decide on warning information and control practices. Therefore, a considerable body of experience exists with these data. The use of acute data should be accompanied by a clear definition of why acute effects impose a health concern, in order not to place too much emphasis on the short-term/high-dose effects if exposures are expected to be at low levels. This question of exposure also has consequences for the choice of relevant data and the choice of any score-aggregation method to be used.

It is important to note that longer-term or chronic effects often do not reflect the responses seen in short-term, higher-level exposures. Conversely, there is no universal way to equate results of acute effect ranking/scoring with ranks or scores for extended-exposure/noncancer effects or carcinogenicity. For this reason, acute health effects scores generally should not be combined with rankings for the other effects categories, unless it becomes necessary to aggregate all 3 into a common index (e.g., toxicity) for screening or basic ranking purposes .

The state of the science is fairly advanced in terms of standardized testing requirements, e.g., those required by the Organization for Economic Cooperation and Development (OECD) or the USEPA. However, there are new tests and testing concepts being developed, such as the limit test for acute toxicity. Because of the trend toward limiting animal testing, Bayesian statistical methods have also been introduced. Similarly, there is a trend in irritation studies to incorporate in vitro tests and possibly replace live animal tests.

A sample list of specific effects for consideration and the methods to measure and quantify these effects are presented in Table 3-1. Although not all-inclusive, these reflect many of the acute toxicity measures for which data are commonly available.

Data issues

Because there is a tremendous diversity in quality and quantity of available data, it is essential to incorporate flexibility into a CRS system. In addition, there are distinct applications for chemical ranking systems, which require different sets of questions to be answered. To accommodate these needs, a tiered approach to chemical scoring is suggested. For acute data, tiers may contain different layers of complexity to cope with different numbers of chemicals to be reviewed. A second type of tiering involves the evaluation of problem-specific or program-specific sectors of effects such as oral toxicity for food additives or dermal irritation for cosmetics and sensitization for occupational exposures.

Minimum data requirements. By design, CRS systems may be applied to chemicals with very little or no epidemiological data and often little experimental data as well. Defining a minimum dataset is application dependent. However, for best application of a scoring system, a minimum dataset should have at least one experimentally derived effect measure. The development of a base set of data (acute lethality, skin and eye irritation) is ideal for such application. Without the universal application of this requirement, data will always be lacking for even the simplest scoring exercise.

Table 3-1 Selected acute health effects and measurements

Effect	Target	Route	Effect measure	Species
Lethality	system	oral	LD50 (n) LD_{Lo} (n) Limit (s) Toxicity class (s)	human rodent rabbit
		dermal	LD50 (n) LD_{Lo} (n) Limit (s) Toxicity class (s)	human rodent rabbit
		inhalation	LC50 (n) LC_{Lo} (n) Limit (s) Toxicity class (s)	human rodent
		parenteral	LD50*	rodent
Incapacitation/ narcotic effect	CNS	inhalation	NOAEL/LOAEL (n) Report (s)	human rodent
			NOAEL/LOAEL (n) Report (s)	
Irritation/ corrosion	skin	skin	Report (s)	human rodent rabbit
			Effect score (s)	
	respiratory tract	inhalation	NOAEL/LOAEL (n)	human rodent
			RD50 (n)	
			Effect score (s) Sensory irritation (n)	
	eye	eye	Report (s)	human rabbit
			Draize test (s)	rabbit
Sensitization	immune	dermal	Patch test (s) Report (s)	human guinea pig
			Maximization (s)	
	immune	inhalation	Report (s)	human rodent

* - if no other data are available
n = numeric dose
s = score

Data availability. Although ideally at least one experimentally derived effect measure should exist for scoring, in reality there often may be situations in which even a minimal body of acute data is not available. In these situations, SAR data may be substituted for measured effect values. It should be noted that SAR is not very well developed for acute effects and is mostly restricted to qualitative statements and/or relative values. Thus, actually measured data generally should be considered more significant than SAR (see section titled "Structure-Activity Relationships"). The use of SAR-derived data should be indicated in any summary report of effects data or scores.

Numeric data measurements versus scored measurements. Traditionally, lethality has been reported in terms of numeric values (full LD50 study), whereas more recent studies focus on scores (toxicity classes). If there is numeric information available, its use is preferable if the data quality allows it. Although numeric values may be aggregated into ranges for scoring, it is preferable to maintain the numeric value for ranking whenever possible.

Aggregation

The simplest form of data aggregation is the conversion of numeric data to a common metric. For low-observed-effects (LD_{Lo} or minimum lethal dose [MLD]) values may be converted to LC50 (lethal concentration to 50% of test population) values by multiplying by a factor of 2. Common spacing factors for dosing acute studies may typically range from 1.5 to 4.

Conversions based on inhalation LC50 values for different exposure times can be performed according to Haber's Law, or a similar conversion formula, for substances with a lung half-life longer than the exposure time. Note however, that these are difficult data to obtain and that particle size plays a major role in deposition and clearance. The rule does not hold for volatile substances that readily attain equilibrium. Haber's Law states that

$$C_xT = k$$

where

C_x	=	concentration of toxicant x,
T	=	time, and
k	=	a constant.

Applying Haber's Law, if a 15-minute exposure to 420 ppm of toxicant x kills 50% of the animals exposed, one could predict that 105 ppm for 1 hour or 26 ppm for 4 hours would also kill 50% of the animals exposed.

Data obtained from different routes of exposure (i.e., LC50 values in mg/L and LD50 [lethal dose to 50% of test population] values in mg/kg) can be converted to equivalent values by applying standardized algorithms that consider inhalation rates, exposure time, and absorption characteristics of the inhaled substances as related to ingestion characteristics. Caution should be used when oral values are converted to inhalation LC50s because the algorithm cannot allow for lung-specific effects.

The ultimate goal is to select the most sensitive of the appropriate endpoints applicable to the ultimate use of the ranking exercise after issues of data quality and relevance are explored. Most ranking/scoring efforts identify endpoints with both numeric and non-numeric data. The only way adequately to incorporate all data into an aggregate acute value is to convert data elements to a common metric. This has the obvious problem of loss of valuable data; however, it has the advantage of allowing simultaneous evaluation and comparison of multiple effects. It is difficult to predict what method will be the most appropriate common measure because this will be dependent on the data and on the underlying purpose of the ranking exercise. However, the goal is to preserve the significance of the actual data available.

Following are 2 examples of scoring systems: Example 3-1 uses a dual numeric score to distinguish clearly actual measured data from those estimated by SAR (Sampaolo and Binetti 1986). Example 3-2 depicts a narrative way of scoring (Gjøs et al. 1989).

Example 3-1 Toxicological Properties
(Sampaolo and Binetti 1986)

Acute toxicity (oral LD50, cutaneous LD50, inhalatory LC50)	Not harmful	0	Whether on the basis of chemical structure or of other acute toxicity data:	
	Harmful	1		
	Toxic	3		
	Very toxic	5	It is possible to exclude acute harmfulness through the 3 absorption routes.	0
			Acute harmfulness is generally suspected.	1
			Acute, not lethal, effects could be expected.	3
			Acute lethal effects could be expected.	5
Skin irritation/corrosion (erythema, and/or edema) and/or eye irritation/corrosion (cornea, iris, conjunctivae) according to the EEC "Guide on classification and labeling"	Negative	0	On the basis of chemical structure:	
	Irritating to skin (score ≥2)	1	It is possible to exclude irritant or corrosive potency.	0
	Corrosive to skin within 4 h	2	There are faint indications of irritant potency.	1
	Irritating to eyes	2	There are evident indications of irritant potency.	2
	Corrosive to skin within 3 min	3	There are evident indications of corrosive potency.	3
			It can be classified as very toxic.	3
Sensitization according to the EEC "Guide on classification and labeling"	Negative	0	On the basis of chemical structure:	
	Positive cutaneously	1	It is possible to exclude sensitization.	0
	Positive by inhalation	2	Information is unavailable.	0.5
			There are generic indications of sensitization.	1
			There are specific indications of sensitization.	2
			It can be classified as very toxic .	3

Example 3-2 Selection Elements for Health Effects
(Gjøs et al. 1989)

Selection element	Low (L)	Medium (M)	High (H)
Acute toxicity LD50 oral, rat (mg/kg)	LD50 > 2000	25 < LD50 ≤ 2000	LD50 ≤ 25
LD50 dermal, rat/rabbit (mg/kg)	LD50 > 2000	50 < LD50 ≤ 2000	LD50 ≤ 50
LC50 inhalation rat (mg/L)*	LC50 > 20	0.5 < LC50 ≤ 20	LC50 ≤ 0.5
Irritation	no effect reported	effect reported	
Sensitization	no effect reported		effect reported

LD50 : median lethal dose
LC50 : median lethal concentration

Total classification of health effects
H : at least one element H
M : at least two elements M
L : data exist on at least 2 elements
? : data exist on only 1 element or no data

* conversion from ppm : mg/L = $\dfrac{MW}{24464}$ ppm

Noncarcinogenic effects due to extended exposures

NOEL, NOAEL, and LOAEL

Detailed studies of effects due to extended exposure commonly include assessments on specific organ systems, including histopathology and clinical chemistry. Testing often includes reproductive and developmental toxicity, neurotoxicity, metabolism, pharmaco-kinetics, and in vitro genotoxicity tests. Sometimes the results of more specialized tests are used, reflecting other responses including immunotoxicity, behavioral effects, and effects on the endocrine system. For each of these areas, numerous protocols are utilized. The studies produce multiple endpoints that are characterized by the type of effect produced, the severity of the effect, the magnitude of the observed changes in the tested individuals, and the proportion of the tested individuals that respond at each dose rate and duration of exposure. The plethora of health effects that may be investigated in epidemiological, clinical, and laboratory studies poses some fundamental problems that must be addressed when designing any CRS system, namely 1) which specific endpoints should be included and 2) how these can be summarized and/or standardized to permit scoring and ranking across many different kinds and severities of effects. There are no set answers to these problems; they must be addressed by the designers of a given CRS system depending on their purpose and the intended application of the results.

Responses to chemical exposures may be classified as

- frank effect levels (FELs), exposures that result in obvious and often relatively severe effects (e.g., pathologic changes with organ disfunction);
- LOAELs, exposures where effects are observed that are considered to be adverse but that may not be severe (e.g., reversible pathologic or enzyme changes);
- NOAELs, exposures where effects are observed but are considered not biologically significant or adverse (e.g., slight changes in body weight, food consumption); or
- NOELs, exposures that produce no observable toxicologic or pharmacologic effect.

The NOAEL and NOEL cluster about the region where the most sensitive effects detectable in the test protocol are beginning to disappear, and the LOAEL usually lies only slightly above these levels. Consequently, these levels are markers of the threshold region, although the LOAEL level may need to be modified to yield the equivalent of an NOAEL. These levels represent the most sensitive effects found in the experimental protocol, and most have exposure units of mg/kg/d for the duration of the test. Inhalation NOAELs and LOAELs, also referred to as NOAECs and LOAECs, may be expressed in terms of mg/m^3 or ppm in air per defined exposure period, continuous or intermittent exposure, e.g., 8 hours or 24 hours for 30 days. For comparison purposes, these may require conversion into mg/kg/d equivalents. An alternative approach comparable in some respects to the NOAEL is the ED10, the dosage rate at which 10% of the organisms respond as determined from a statistical dose-response model. At the 10% level, the choice of the dose-response model is not very critical, because the log-probit, log-logit, or the maximum likelihood estimate (MLE) solution of the multistage models will give similar estimates of the 10th percentile. The 10th percentile has often been selected because it represents an incidence of responses that is near the threshold of resolution for specific effects in most chronic toxicity studies and is generally within the experimental range.

The NOELs, NOAELs, and LOAELs are influenced more by the content of the testing protocol (i.e., the number and complexity of parameters measured) than by the duration of dosing once this extends beyond 21 to 30 days. Exceptions to this are substances that require longer to reach toxicokinetic equilibrium or that produce carcinogenic responses. Therefore, in most instances, this metric can be used as a common basis for comparison of the chronic toxicities of many substances. This approach summarizes important aspects of the dose-response relationships for sensitive responses after extended exposures. Depending on the requirements of the ranking system, it may be necessary to convert an LOAEL to an NOAEL where an actual NOAEL value may not exist. Typically, a 10-fold adjustment has been used to lower the LOAEL dose to the range expected to demonstrate no adverse effects (e.g., in the USEPA RfD methodology). The NOEL/NOAEL data allow an initial ordinal ranking of the toxicities of individual substances in units that are related to dose rates. It should be noted that a similar approach is taken in most of the extant ranking and scoring systems, though often using a further step of converting dose units to arbitrary scores and discarding the original data early in the analysis. Such conversions to scores, which typically represent ranges of effect levels, make it more complicated and potentially less accurate to incorporate exposure data into the ranking and scoring framework.

Data availability for extended exposure effects

The amount of toxicological information that is available for specific compounds can vary from a total absence of toxicological studies to minimal acute studies to complex studies reported in extensive detail. For datasets where only LOAEL values may be found, it may be reasonable to adjust these values to a surrogate NOAEL by lowering the LOAEL by 1 dosage unit or by 1 order of magnitude or by application of benchmark dose techniques. When there are no subchronic/chronic NOELs, NOAELs, or LOAELs, there are methods that allow the estimation of values at or below actual NOAEL values from use of acute toxicity values (Weil and McCollister 1963; Weil et al. 1969; McNamara 1971; Venman and Flaga 1985; Layton et al. 1987). There are new versions of quantitative structure-activity relationship (QSAR) models, such as the TOPKAT computer model (Health Designs, Inc. 1990), that construct estimates of LOAEL values from structure alone. This allows comparisons to be made among a wide array of compounds. Further discussion of the use of SARs follows in the section titled "Minimum data discussion." It is clear, however, that the quality and reliability of such derived values will differ, and therefore it will be very important to have an indicator of quality to accompany the data, e.g., very high (VH), high (H), moderate (M), low (L), or very low (VL). The section titled "Modifiers" addresses data quality issues and how such modifiers may be defined and applied.

Aggregation

Chemical ranking systems for human health effects from extended exposures may be based upon arrays of various regulatory limits or criteria, such as

- DWELs (drinking water exposure limits, USEPA);
- RfDs (reference doses, USEPA);
- RfCs (reference concentrations in air, USEPA);
- PELs (permissible exposure limits in air, U.S. Health Education and Welfare [USHEW]); and
- TLVs (threshold limit values in air, American Conference of Governmental Industrial Hygienists [ACGIH]).

However, these regulatory limits often differ significantly among administrative units, i.e., depending on whether their purpose is to protect drinking water quality versus occupational health. They may include factors other than health (e.g., economics), analytical, and treatment capabilities. The toxicity data are usually subjected to extensive manipulation to attain the desired degrees of safety in the course of developing exposure limits, i.e., through the application of uncertainty factors and exposure assumptions. Furthermore, the number of chemicals for which such values exist is limited. In contrast, CRS systems are not intended for classical risk assessments. They are not designed to be protective and therefore need not reflect the variety of risk assessment methods that are inherent in recommended exposure levels of regulatory limits. Therefore, the initial ranking/scoring for human health should be designed to preserve the actual experimental data as far as possible in the process.

The ideal initial outcome of the ranking of chemicals for health effects after extended exposures would be a list of chemicals ranked according to their basic NOEL/NOAEL values, including a data quality identifier that should be retained in the final report. Thus the initial ranking could be as follows:

Chemical	NOEL/NOAEL (mg/kg/d)	Data quality
XChem	0.02	Moderate
YChem	0.7	Very high
ZChem	2	Low

If the original question that lead to the CRS exercise was fairly simple, this could be the final output. However, it may be important to consider severity, pharmacokinetics, genotoxicity, or a number of additional factors, depending upon the basic screening and ranking question that has been asked. In such cases, it may be necessary to modify the original ranking, depending upon the strength of the modifying factors.

Although it is preferable to retain the use of chemical-specific NOELs, NOAELs, or LOAELs for some ranking uses, it may be necessary to aggregate NOELs, NOAELs, or LOAELs into simple groupings or cluster ranges. Such aggregate clusters may be defined by either a narrative or numeric value. Examples of 2 scoring systems currently in use, the UCSS (USEPA 1993a) (Example 3-3) and the Canadian Accelerated Reduction/Elimination of Toxics (ARET) Scoring System (Environment Canada and Ontario Ministry of the Environment and Energy [OMOEE] 1994) (Example 3-4) are included here for review.

Example 3-3 UCSS Human Health Hazard Scoring Table – Noncancer Effects (USEPA 1993a)

Data element	High (3)	Medium (2)	Low (1)
		Ranking	
Level 1 data elements			
Chronic NOAEL	< 0.1 mg/kg/d	0.1–10 mg/kg/d	> 10 mg/kg/d
Chronic LOAEL	< 1 mg/kg/d	1–100 mg/kg/d	> 100 mg/kg/d
Subchronic NOAEL	< 1 mg/kg/d	1–100 mg/kg/d	> 100 mg/kg/d
Subchronic LOAEL	10 mg/kg/d	10–1000 mg/kg/d	> 1000 mg/kg/d
Level 2 data elements			
Structure-Activity Team (SAT) calls	High	Medium–High, Medium	Low–Medium, Low

Example 3-4 ARET Scoring Criteria
(OMOEE 1994)

Element name	Endpoint and units	0	2	4	6	8	10
Acute lethality	oral LD50 (mg/kg)	> 5000	> 500–5000	> 50–500	> 5–50	> 0.5–5	≤ 0.5
	dermal LD50 (mg/mg)	> 5000	> 500–5000	> 50–500	> 5–50	> 0.5–5	≤ 0.5
	inhal LC50 (mg/m^3)	> 15000	> 1500–15000	> 150–1500	> 15–150	> 1.5–15	≤ 1.5
	aquatic LC 50 (mg/L)	> 1000	> 100–1000	> 10–100	> 1–10	> 0.1–1	≤ 0.1
Chronic/ sub-chronic toxicity, non-mammals	aquatic						
	EC50 (mg/L)	≥ 20	2 – < 20	0.2 – <2	0.02 – < 0.2	< 0.02*	< 0.02*
	MATC (mg/L)	≥ 2	0.2 – < 2	0.02 – < 0.2	0.002 – < 0.02	< 0.002*	< 0.002*
	NOAEC (mg/L)	≥ 0.2	0.02 – < 0.2	0.002 – < 0.02	0.0002 – < 0.002	< 0.0002*	< 0.0002*
	terrestrial						
	subchronic (NOEL mg/kg/d)	≥ 1000	100 – < 1000	10 – < 100	1 – < 10	< 1*	< 1*
	chronic (NOEL mg/kg/d)	≥ 500	50 – < 500	5 – < 50	0.5 – < 5	< 0.5* *in one genus	< 0.5* *in different genera
Chronic/ sub-chronic toxicity, plants (water, mg/L) (air, mg/m^3) (soil, mg/kg)	% growth reduction: ≤ 5 (= NOEL)						
	water	> 10	> 1–10	> 0.1–1	> 0.01–0.1	0.001–0.01	< 0.001
	air	> 100	> 10–100	> 1–10	> 0.1–1	0.01–0.1	< 0.01
	soil	> 100	> 10–100	> 1–10	> 0.1–1	0.01–0.1	< 0.01
	> 5–50 (= EC50)						
	water	> 100	> 10–100	> 1–10	> 0.1–1	0.01–0.1	< 0.01
	air	> 1000	> 100–1000	> 10–100	> 1–10	0.1–1	< 0.1
	soil	> 1000	> 100–1000	> 10–100	> 1–10	0.1–1	< 0.1
	> 50						
	water	> 1000	> 100–1000	> 10–100	> 1–10	0.1–1	< 0.1
	air	> 10000	> 1000–10000	> 100–1000	> 10–100	1–10	< 1
	soil	> 10000	> 1000–10000	> 100–1000	> 10–100	1–10	< 1
Chronic/ sub-chronic toxicity, mammals [1]	oral NOEL (mg/kg/d)	> 1000	> 100–1000	> 10–100	> 1–10	> 0.1–1	≤ 0.1
	inhal NOEL (mg/m^3)	> 3000	> 300–3000	> 30–300	> 3–30	> 0.3–3	≤ 0.3

[1] Criteria based on studies of ≥90-d duration. If only shorter-term subchronic studies are available, NOEL is divided by 5 prior to scoring for toxicity.

Carcinogenic effects

Carcinogen classification

Chemical carcinogens present unique challenges for CRS for a variety of reasons. In most current risk assessments for this effect, it is generally assumed that carcinogenicity is a nonthreshold process, i.e., that there is some probability of tumor development at any level of exposure. Consequently, the default methods generally applied to cancer risk estimates do not recommend the calculation of a dose or concentration below which this effect will not occur, as is generally done for other types of adverse effects. As a better understanding of mechanisms and the influence of pharmacokinetics in the carcinogenic process of various compounds develops, the nonthreshold concept may change, at least for some substances. However, detailed evaluation of the weight of evidence for carcinogenicity (i.e., consideration of such factors as dose-response relationships, the specific tumor types produced, the likely mechanisms of carcinogenicity, the validity of extrapolation between species, etc.) is beyond the scope of most CRS applications.

Instead, in some chemical ranking methods, carcinogenicity is evaluated on the basis of classification schemes developed by the International Agency for Research on Cancer (IARC 1987), the USEPA (1997b), or the European Union (EU). In these schemes, which are used throughout the world, the evidence that a substance is carcinogenic based on epidemiological studies, animal bioassays, and other supporting data is classified into one of several groups using established criteria. Appropriate use of published classification systems in scoring carcinogenic effects can reflect a general level of concern for the chemicals being considered. Although the simple classification schemes ignore potency and probable exposure levels, this approach supports simple evaluations of a large number of carcinogenic chemicals, which are readily accessible and which can easily be reviewed and understood.

Another method applied to carcinogenic effects involves developing "potency" factors for use in ranking of chemicals. In this approach, estimates of the specific dose of the chemical that would cause a defined incidence of response (e.g., the ED10 or the slope factor) are calculated. (The slope factor is an upper bound estimate of the probability of an individual developing cancer from a lifetime exposure to a carcinogen. The ED10 is the concentration or dose that, when experienced over the lifetime, induces a 10% increase in the incidence of tumors considered to be associated with exposure.) USEPA's (1997b) Integrated Risk Information System (IRIS) and Health Effects Assessment Summary Tables (HEAST) databases (USEPA 1995b) provide cancer potency slopes for some carcinogens. The USEPA (1996) draft Guidelines for Carcinogen Risk Assessment recommended use of the ED10 approach as a default unless available information precludes its use. However, there are many other substances for which there is some evidence of carcinogenicity but for which published estimates of these values are not readily available. Although ED10 values may be calculated for many of these substances, in order to develop such data the chemical must have been tested, the proper study and endpoint in the study must be identified, and the correct response value must be selected. Development of ED10 values or potency estimates for a large number of substances would probably exceed the resources and technical expertise available to most scoring and ranking applications.

Availability of carcinogenicity data

For many chemicals, human epidemiological studies will not be available to assess carcinogenic potential (and indeed, may not be possible to conduct). Evaluation will then have to be based upon animal bioassay data. In such instances, if the data from animal bioassays are sufficiently strong, it is desirable that the weight given to these data be similar to the weights given to substances for which the scores are based on data from studies in humans. Unfortunately, there are thousands of chemicals in commerce for which human epidemiological and animal bioassay data are not available upon which to judge carcinogenic potential. It is important that any scoring system for this effect not merely reflect the completeness of the database. Therefore, an SAR should be used whenever possible to account for lack of actual data. Because of the perceived importance of carcinogenicity in evaluating a chemical's adverse effects, the SAR for this endpoint is the best developed of the 3 areas of human health effects considered here (see section titled "Structure-activity relationships for carcinogenicity").

Aggregation of carcinogenicity data

In some chemical ranking applications, the classification schemes used by such agencies as the IARC and the USEPA are combined with a measure of carcinogenic potency, usually the slope factor or the ED10. The inclusion of information on both the weight of evidence for carcinogenicity and the potency to induce cancer is desirable because a dose somewhat comparable to the noncancer NOEL or NOAEL in mg/kg/d may be established as well as a judgment made on the weight of evidence for carcinogenicity in humans. This approach places carcinogenicity on a more equal footing with noncancer endpoints, a situation that has not always been the case.

Because of the problems earlier identified in ability to obtain ED10 values, it is suggested that most CRS schemes be based on the classification of substances by IARC and USEPA, modified where possible by the ED10. For a general ranking and scoring system, it is considered preferable to use the ED10 to express carcinogenic potency, as opposed to such quantities as the slope factor because the ED10 is within or close to the observed effects range. This avoids the numerous uncertainties associated with low-dose extrapolation. Two systems that rely on the use of both the quantitative ED10 and qualitative weight of evidence, the UCSS (USEPA 1993a) and a system developed by Foran and Glenn (1993), are included as Examples 3-5 and 3-6.

Example 3-5: Human Health Hazard Scoring – Cancer
(USEPA 1993a)

Data element	Weight of evidence	Ranking High (3)	Medium (2)	Low (1)
Level 1 data elements				
Reportable quantity (RQ) potency factor (1 / ED10)	A or B	> 10 mg/kg/d	0.2–10 mg/kg/d	< 0.2 mg/kg/d
RQ potency factor (1 / ED10)	C or Unknown	> 80 mg/kg/d	1–80 mg/kg/d	< 1 mg/kg/d
Level 2 data elements				
Structure Activity Team (SAT) Call	Any	High	Medium–High, Medium	Low–Medium, Low

Example 3-6: Classification and Scoring Scheme for Carcinogenicity
(Foran and Glenn 1993)

Weight of evidence
(WOE) group	Definition
A	Sufficient evidence of cancer in humans, or
B	evidence of cancer in 2 or more laboratory animal species or strains, or replicate studies, and
C	evidence of cancer in 1 laboratory animal species, or benign tumors only, or
D	inadequate data suggest carcinogenic potential, or no data.

Potency group	1/ ED10 *
1	> 100
2	1–100
3	< 1

* 1 / ED10 is the potency factor used to assign reportable quantities for carcinogens by the CERCLA Section 102 program. ED10 is the dose (mg/kg/d) calculated to result in 10% tumor incidence.

		Potency group 1	2	3
	A	H	H	M
WOE	B	H	M	L
group	C	M	L	L
	D	No hazard ranking		

It should be noted that the classification of the USEPA is a weight-of-evidence scheme that is more risk-based than other classification systems, whereas more substances have been evaluated by the IARC. In instances where a substance has not been evaluated by these agencies but epidemiological or experimental studies of its carcinogenicity are available, the criteria used by these agencies may be used to classify and score the compound. As with the noncancer effects, it is desirable to rank chemicals relatively, using the actual data for the given effect, and to carry that data as far as possible in the ranking process. If it becomes necessary to group or cluster values and assign arbitrary weight, Examples 3-5 and 3-6 demonstrate aggregation and weighting based on both a numeric and narrative value.

Modifiers

Modifiers are factors that cannot be directly related to relative hazard in a quantitative fashion. They are factors that require professional judgment and, because of their subjective nature, represent a source of disparity observed between existing CRS protocols. Depending upon the chemical being compared, modifiers may indicate that consideration of measurable effects alone does not adequately represent differences in potential hazard between 2 chemicals. Modifiers may be used to represent these differences or necessary adjustments on measures of potential hazard. Possible points of influence of modifiers and their relationship to the entire human health assessment ranking process is identified in Figure 3-1.

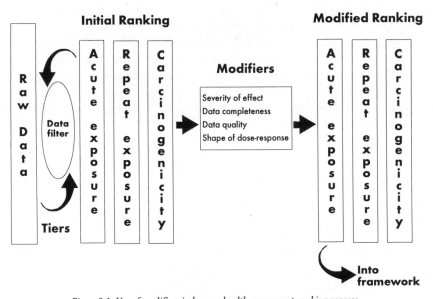

Figure 3-1 Use of modifiers in human health assessment ranking process

Modifiers that have been identified as being important in the evaluation of chemical hazards include the following:

- Data quality and quantity
  - quality of the data used to derive effect category scores (i.e., NOAEL for subchronic/chronic noncancer effects and scores for carcinogenicity and acute toxicity)
  - extent to which the chemical has been tested (data completeness)
- Severity of effect
  - spectrum/gradient of effects
  - shape of the dose-response curve for the effect being considered (i.e., potency)
- Potential for mutagenic or genotoxic effects

Each of these modifiers may or may not significantly affect the category score or ranking, depending on the specific chemicals and data being considered and on the purpose of a given CRS system.

Data quality and quantity

The level of confidence associated with the scoring system and ranking of any group of chemicals will largely reflect the completeness and quality of the dataset being considered. Chemicals that have been tested extensively for a wide range of potential effects need to be distinguished from those with limited testing data. Similarly, the quality of the individual studies used to derive effect scores must be considered and reflected. Where data are missing and extrapolation methods are used to fill information gaps, the error associated with these methods must be considered.

Uncertainty in toxicology evaluations is inherent because of variability across species, study durations, and multiple and often widely spaced dose levels. This requires careful technical evaluation before use of any data and reflection of this uncertainty in effect assessment.

No absolute minimum dataset has been considered necessary. However, depending on the design of the CRS, the absence of experimental data in a key category may preclude a thorough evaluation due to inadequate or insufficient information. To establish some prediction of effect, for instance, it may be possible to extrapolate across categories, i.e., acute and chronic data. For example, if exact acute data are not available but a longer term study has been conducted showing NOAELs at dose levels higher than the acute dose levels of concern, there may be, in fact, no acute toxicity concern warranted for the substance. Some attempts have been made to extrapolate from acute to chronic data, but further research is needed in this area, and the use of extrapolation should be moderated by its potential high degree of uncertainty. For screening purposes, SAR evaluations also require estimations of uncertainty, and those estimates must be noted.

Severity of effect

The screening of health effects should consider a broad spectrum of effects, including systemic and target organ toxicity and specific effects of interest such as reproductive and developmental toxicity. The use of the NOEL or NOAEL for noncancer effects is considered the desirable way to reflect the inherent toxicity of a chemical. However, the diversity of effects that may be reported in multiple animal or human studies may lead to comparisons of effects that differ dramatically in their potential to cause long-term harm.

For example, to compare and rank the potential hazards of 2 chemicals with similar NOAELs, it will be valuable and necessary to consider the severity of the effects represented by the NOAELs. An NOAEL derived for an effect such as transient upper respiratory tract irritation is not directly comparable to one representing permanent peripheral nervous system damage. Alternatively, another comparison of severity may involve 2 chemicals with significantly different NOAELs, which differ inversely in the severity of effects. For example, chemical A may exhibit an NOAEL for the most sensitive effect that is relatively high (indicating a low hazard), but the effect observed is severe (e.g., lung damage). Chemical B exhibits a much lower NOAEL (i.e., greater hazard) but for an effect that is much less severe (e.g., skin irritation).

These cases require more detailed information and evaluation if they are to be resolved with any degree of confidence. Depending upon the final intended use of the specific ranking and scoring exercise, the conclusions of ranking these compounds may need to be modified to reflect the importance of the severity of effect. Other critical information that may be considered in defining the final ranking position between 2 chemicals include these:

- gradient of responses observed;
- results of short-term or in vitro tests;
- pharmacokinetics;
- molecular action and pathology;
- SARs;
- preclinical effects indicators;
- number of experimental species exhibiting effects;
- various routes of administration;
- different dose regimens;
- epidemiologic data;
- dose-response gradient;
- high incidence rate, large excess risk;
- high level of statistical significance in relevant studies; and
- temporal relationship of the association.

Genotoxicity/mutagenicity

For most CRS applications, the results of genotoxicity tests are considered to be useful primarily for the interpretation of potential mechanisms of carcinogenicity or teratogenicity. Genotoxicity or mutagenicity may be considered a measure of increased concern (i.e., genotoxic versus nongenotoxic effects) or may be useful as an indicator of, or supporting data for, carcinogenicity or teratogenicity (i.e., a flag for carcinogenic or teratogenic potential) when direct data from long-term studies or epidemiology studies are limited or unavailable for a chemical. When this information is used as a modifier, it may be useful to consider the weight of evidence for genotoxicity by giving more weight to genotoxic effects observed for in vivo test systems, to genotoxic effects observed in mammalian cells, and to direct tests of mutagenicity as compared with indicator tests.

Structure for Assessing Health Effects in CRS

Key process elements

It is important to note that the use of health effects data proposed here is not for risk assessment purposes or the setting of safety factors. The application of data as described is intended only for classification, ranking, and/or prioritization of chemicals on the basis of relative measures of their toxicities.

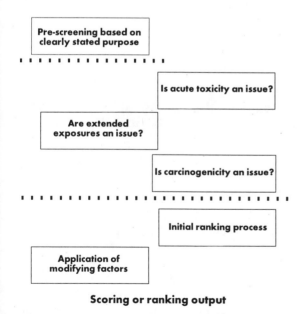

Figure 3-2 Key elements of assessing health effects and their relationships

The key elements of the process and their relation to each other are identified in Figure 3-2. Although the system is designed to be uncomplicated, a full complement of available data on a chemical (including evaluation of acute lethality, sensitization, irritation, neurotoxicity, immunotoxicity, reproductive and developmental effects, other subchronic and chronic system or organ toxicity, as well as carcinogenicity) may be utilized, depending on the purpose for which the scoring system is intended and the availability of data. All available data should be considered for use, with a preference given for human effects or epidemiologic data. Animal data may be used in cases where epidemiologic data do not exist or are of inadequate quality or extent to characterize effects in humans. Structure-activity team (SAT) estimations may be used where data are missing or of such poor quality as to be unusable. It must be recognized that the quality of SAR estimates also varies.

Tiered approach

The intended purpose or use of the screening system should establish the need for (and extent of review necessary for) specific categories, subcategories, and/or specific effects prior to conducting the screen. Users of the data may elect to look at all or a subset of the data, creating in effect a customized tier of data applicable to their own use. In reality, tiers of review are usually limited by available resources (time and manpower), by data quality and/or quantity, by the specific effects of interest or the severity of effect, and by the need to limit the size of the universe of chemicals for consideration.

Tiered reviews are typically constructed based on consideration of limited datasets and effects. For instance, a first tier review might accommodate an application in which chemicals are prioritized for future activities, such as testing, substitution, or reduction. For this example, there may be minimal data available and a large universe of chemicals to address. A simple listing of available data may reveal datasets with only acute oral LD50 values, irritation studies, and mutagenicity screening data. After the review is conducted, there may be a need for a second tier screen of chemicals selected from the first tier using a more in-depth data analysis. Data used for this review might include thorough evaluation of subchronic study endpoints to determine NOELs or NOAELs for the chemicals. These chemicals may be further rank-adjusted by consideration of the type and severity of effects noted, along with the presence or absence of positive mutagenicity data.

A final tier might be used to further evaluate the chemicals defined via tier 2 for consideration for full, detailed hazard assessment. More extensive data evaluation would be warranted. Data review might include carcinogenicity, reproductive and developmental effects, neuro- and immunotoxicity assessment, along with any other subchronic/chronic adverse effects. Relative rankings of these compounds might be modified by multiple effects noted, critical reproductive effects noted, or the dose-response and weight of evidence noted for carcinogenicity.

These examples should be considered on a continuum of possible applications, and therefore, it is expected that there can be many tiers between scoring outcomes. Given the diversity in data quality and quantity available, it is essential to incorporate flexibility into the screening and scoring process to allow a "best fit" with the resources available, to clarify the purpose of the screening activity, and to best utilize available data. Tiers can be established based on arbitrary decisions about minimum data requirements, which may be necessary to drive data development. However, tiered minimum data requirements are not recommended when one is forced to conduct screening and scoring exercises utilizing only the data at hand. Efforts should be focused on utilizing as much of the available data as possible.

Data Requirements

General principles

The data presented in a ranking/scoring system are generally of heterogeneous quality and relevance. If there is more than one value available for any given effect, or if there are data on effects closely related to each other (i.e., differing in species or application route only), a choice has to be made about which data to use. The following suggestions are made to address the most common situations within individual effects.

Data quality

Available data for effects vary in quality from highly reliable, comprehensive studies to marginal observations taken from unpublished studies that cannot be reviewed. In addition, although many results are reported in summary literature and on material safety data sheets (MSDSs), the raw data generally cannot be obtained nor assessed. Many older studies in the published literature may have used a large number of animals, but were not conducted under good laboratory practices (GLPs). More recent studies have an improved quality by adhering to GLP guidelines, while their reduced number of animals limits their weight of evidence. In a situation where multiple studies report the same effect, the GLP data are considered highest quality and should be selected over other reports.

Carefully conducted and reported animal toxicity studies may conflict with human studies, which may be of doubtful quality and may rely on case reports and other nonstandardized methods. Although human data are of greater relevance, in instances where questions about the quality of these data exist, it must be carefully decided whether these data still should be considered of primary importance.

Number of studies/choice of studies

There are many situations where a single endpoint will be reported in multiple studies. In these situations there are several options. The first two could be applied "mechanically" 1) to average numerical values or average reported scores, or 2) to take the most sensitive reported values or most sensitive, plausible reported values. The best option is to select a single reported effect based on relevance of species, route, and GLP considerations, but this requires some expert judgment. The options selected and the criteria used in applying expert judgment should be explicitly stated.

Conflicting scoring systems. Often summary data or scored data are the only data available to evaluate. Implicit in these scoring systems are individual judgments that may not be transparent. Problems would exist in tracing these judgments back to the original data.

An effect reported by using a summary value that provides the most transparent process should be the best choice.

Relevance/choice of species. Whenever possible, data for the most relevant species (human) should be used. If these are missing and there is a choice of other species, the one most widely used for the type of test should be chosen for the sake of comparability (e.g., rat for acute oral, rabbit for eye, etc.)

Relevance of route. If there is a choice of routes, the most sensitive one generally should be taken, with the exception that parenteral application should be omitted due to lack of relevance when other routes are available. This rule may be overridden, of course, if the purpose of the ranking/scoring study clearly indicates that a given route should be given preference (e.g., oral for screening food additives, inhalation or dermal for worker exposures).

Relevance of effect

If multiple effects are reported, possible options are to choose the most sensitive effect or the one most relevant for the purpose of the ranking/scoring study. For example, for accidents and spills in the ambient environment, the key effect may be lethality, whereas for the workplace environment, irritation/corrosion, sensitization, or longer-term systemic effects may be more appropriate.

Minimum data discussion

A concise but informative toxicity profile of a chemical is provided by a dataset containing data on acute toxicity, repeated dose toxicity, and cancer response. Too much information is lost if individual scores in these broad effects areas are combined. Ideally then, a minimum dataset for a chemical should contain data for each of these areas, such as a test of acute lethality, a repeated dose study providing an NOAEL or LOAEL, and a weight-of-evidence determination on carcinogenicity. In reality, even this minimal dataset is available for only a limited number of chemicals, and surrogate data will be needed to fill the data gaps. For some classes of chemicals, missing data may be calculated from other data, e.g., NOAEL from LD50, potential carcinogenicity from SAR, etc. Additional research on predictive or extrapolative methods relevant to human health effects is needed to help fill in some of these data gaps. Scoring system development needs to incorporate sufficient flexibility to recognize this reality and not penalize chemicals for the presence of data while untested chemicals are rewarded for lack of data.

To screen a chemical or list of chemicals for potential human health effects, there are really no minimum data requirements beyond chemical structure. With a structure alone, or perhaps accompanied by some physical–chemical properties, panels of experts such as USEPA's SAT can qualitatively predict effects in each of the areas of acute toxicity, cancer, and noncancer effects. There are also commercially available computer programs (e.g., TOPKAT [Health Designs Inc. 1990], CASE system [Klopman 1984], DEREK system [Lewis et al. 1993]) that will provide a quantitative estimate of acute or sub-chronic toxicity based on structural information alone for some classes of chemicals.

Depending upon the specific application, the tests included in a minimum dataset may vary considerably. Scoring on the basis of SARs may be acceptable for purposes of screening a large number of chemicals, especially if additional assessment is contemplated for chemicals selected by the scoring process. In instances where regulatory or business decisions hinge on the outcome of the scoring exercise, a minimum set of actual toxicity data would be most desirable.

Whether a chemical's scores are based primarily on SARs, on actual data, or on a mixture of the two, the basis of the individual scores should reflect the appropriate measure of uncertainty in the data that accompanies the score through any further manipulations.

Structure-activity relationships

Structure-activity relationship analysis involves the structural analogy of a chemical for which test data are available to an untested chemical that, together with physical–chemical properties, results in a prediction of the potential toxicity of the untested chemical. It is not meant to replace data or to be a substitute for testing. However, when used in concert with available data, it is a valuable tool for flagging chemicals that may present potential hazards for humans. Various SAR systems have been developed that use both quantitative and qualitative estimation techniques. This section will discuss the use of SARs to fill data gaps in scoring systems for 3 categories: acute toxicity, effects of extended exposure, and carcinogenicity. A discussion of the application of SARs for ecological and aquatic effects appears in Chapter 4, "Use of Quantitative Structure-Activity Relationships."

Structure-activity relationships for acute effects

Because acute toxicity data are generally perceived as either readily available or easily attainable, the SARs for these effects are not well developed. It is possible, however, to qualitatively estimate a number of the acute effects by considering the chemical class to which the chemical belongs or by considering the moieties of known toxicity contained in the chemical structure. These estimations most probably would take the form of relative rankings. For example, the oral LD50 value for a chemical with a cyano group that has the potential to be released would be expected to be lower than a chemical where the group would not be expected to be released, although the absolute value could not be estimated. If a sufficient number of analogues existed, bounding estimates could be applied. If qualitative descriptors are used (such as low, moderate, or high), these could be converted to bounding estimates by any number of schemes available from classic toxicology texts, or one could construct a scheme that serves a particular need. One such scheme, used in the USEPA/EU SAR/Minimum Premarket Dataset (MPD) study (USEPA 1994d) to convert qualitative descriptors for acute toxicity into bounding values, is presented below:

Concern level	Oral LD50 (mg/kg)
Low	≥ 2000
Low-moderate	≥ 1000 to < 2000
Moderate	≥ 500 to < 1000
Moderate-high	≥ 50 to < 500
High	< 50

This scheme is presented only as an example; the chemicals of concern in this case were industrial chemicals, and as a class, they were not expected to be particularly acutely toxic. If the chemicals that are being scored are all expected to be of moderate toxicity, then a ranking system should be devised that separates the levels of toxicity with greater resolution.

Skin and eye irritation may also be qualitatively predicted by considering the chemical class. Additionally, chemical reactivity can be an indicator of the potential for irritation to both skin and eyes. However, there are a number of chemicals that may be skin irritants but not eye irritants or vice versa. The state of SARs is not developed to the extent that a distinction between the two can be made. Sensitization may also be predicted by chemical class, i.e., isocyanates have the potential for respiratory sensitization. Other moieties or physical–chemical properties such as molecular weight (MW) may mitigate the concern, but again the SAR is not well understood. Both irritation and sensitization would most likely take the form of "yes/no" predictions.

Structure-activity relationships for extended exposure

Because repeated dose studies are not, in general, perceived as being readily available on the majority of chemicals, the SARs for these effects are better developed. A number of available commercial systems attempt to predict multiple target organ toxicities both quantitatively and qualitatively. Some systems are more transparent than others, allowing the user to judge the quality of the prediction. On the other hand, the nontransparent systems can make reliable predictions if their databases contain many chemicals that are analogous to the ones that are being scored.

Structure-activity relationships for repeated dose toxicity generally depend upon data for the chemical class to which the chemical or chemicals belong, data for analogous chemicals, and known toxicity of various chemical moieties. In some cases, mechanisms of toxicity may be known, but in the vast majority of cases, analog data are used and the mechanism is at best only poorly understood. Again, systems may be inter-converted between qualitative and quantitative by using bounding estimates, although for repeated dose toxicity there are the additional problems of multiple target organs, severity of effects, and seriousness of effects. These issues need to be addressed in any conversion. The scheme used for converting the 28-day repeated dose study results to qualitative terms in the USEPA/EU SAR/MPD study (USEPA 1994d) is shown in Table 3-2.

Table 3-2 Qualitative concern levels for repeated-dose toxicity

Concern level	Criteria
Low	No system toxicity (NOAELs 1 g/kg or greater); or only liver and/or kidney increased organ weight or clinical chemistry changes; LOAELs of >500 mg/kg
Moderate	Organ pathology (micro or gross) with LOAELs of 500 mg/kg or less; clinical chemistry changes and organ weight changes at <500 mg/kg; NOAELs <100 mg/kg
High	Death, organ pathology (micro or gross), multiple organ toxicity; NOAELs <10 mg/kg

This scheme is not meant to be definitive but only to illustrate how the conversion may be accomplished. It should be noted that for this research effort, there were no doses between 500 mg/kg and 1000 mg/kg. The USEPA/EU workgroup knew what dosage levels they were dealing with and adjusted the scale to fit the data. This is not normally the case in most ranking exercises. Therefore, an interval to address NOAELs between 100 mg/kg and 1000 mg/kg (i.e., a moderately low level of concern) must be developed.

Structure-activity relationships for carcinogenicity

Because carcinogenicity historically has been perceived as the most serious endpoint, the SAR for this effect is the best developed of the 3 categories of effects considered here. Numerous systems exist for predicting the carcinogenic potential of chemicals. Unlike the other categories, mechanisms of action are thought to be understood for at least some carcinogens. Systems, again, may be qualitative or quantitative, and classes of known carcinogens play an important role in the prediction process. However, for this effect, SARs have been elucidated that take into account substitutions on the molecule and the activation/deactivation potential of such substitutions for some of the chemical classes. The general principles used in SARs for carcinogenicity predictions are these: ability to reach target site; activation or ability to be activated near or at the target site; and reasonable lifetime of the active chemical to allow interaction with target macromolecules, to display selective, specific, and persistent interaction with target macromolecules, and to affect various stages of carcinogenesis. Consideration of the activating/deactivating factors provide the basis for predicting potential carcinogenic activity.

An expert system under development at USEPA is a computerized attempt to incorporate the logic and knowledge of USEPA experts in deducing whether a chemical has the potential to be carcinogenic. This system is being constructed on a chemical class basis, and its output is a justification report that not only gives a qualitative concern level but also outlines the logic train upon which the level is based. Such a system allows the user to see the rationale used and to make his or her own evaluation of the scheme.

Guiding Principles for Health Effects in CRS

System development

Chemical ranking and scoring activities are conducted for a host of purposes, and it would be impossible to create one particular scoring system that would fit all potential uses. Some examples include evaluating potential health effects of new consumer products, employee protection concerns from process chemicals, community impacts of both sudden and uncontrolled chemical releases, and long-term low-level emissions and discharges. A suite of critical effects elements should be identified from which one could choose specific categories and subcategories of adverse effects to a health effects assessment protocol appropriate to the end use. Therefore, it is critical that the intent of each CRS be clearly defined before initiating the screening effort and that the system be pretested using benchmark chemicals with known properties or concerns to ensure that it will function properly for the intended purpose. Exposure assessment is not directly incorporated into the health effects review but directly influences the design and the calibration of the system, depending on its specific application.

Guiding principles for system development include the following:
- Common categories and subcategories that are important to multiple-purpose systems should be used.
- Inputs and decision-making processes should be simple to use.
- Category endpoints should be transferable directly to more complicated risk assessment activities, unencumbered as much as possible by value judgments or safety factors.
- Outputs should contribute to relative ranking but be value-neutral as to risk or safety.

Aggregation and weighting of human health effects scores

Three basic categories of health effects are discussed in the screening model: acute, sub-chronic/chronic effects, and carcinogenicity. All are considered important for the full evaluation of potential for adverse health effects from exposure. Each of these categories may be equally important, depending on the question that the screening system is designed to answer. Most current ranking/scoring systems arbitrarily assign values and aggregate effects with little attention to the validity of either the individual or aggregate scores. For this reason, the actual endpoint data in mg/kg/d should be used as extensively as possible in the system to preserve the actual data. Further, it generally makes little sense to aggregate acute and extended exposure effects because they are seldom relevant to each other.

For many applications, acute effects may be considered less important in a screen than longer term effects because low-level environmental releases would rarely be in the range of exposures that could lead to acute toxic effects. Knowledge of an acute hazard requires warning information and control practices to prevent immediate toxicity. Thus, exposure to acute levels in an occupational setting tends to be self-limiting or highly controlled by engineering or personal protective equipment. However, direct consumer use, transportation, and accidental spill potential are cases where the acute effects must be considered from a different perspective and perhaps given more weight than data from longer term exposures.

Future Needs and Recommendations

The evolution of CRS will parallel advances in toxicological research, improved exposure measurements, and policy initiatives. As these areas develop, refinements in CRS are expected. Briefly described here are some of the areas of human health research in which changes can be expected in the near future.

1) As the demand for reduced animal testing increases, new methods to evaluate acute toxicity will be developed. As the methods develop, it is critical to determine the relationship between conventional studies in a way that allows the comparable utilization of new methods. Research to develop these relationships will facilitate the incorporation of these new methods into ranking/scoring systems.

2) Currently, new in vitro methods to assess specific endpoints such as skin and eye irritation, teratogenicity, etc., are being developed that by design will reduce the need for animal testing. As methods development proceeds, it must be decided when to incorporate these new methods into ranking/screening systems. Research in the development of these methods should run parallel with studies that correlate these data and validate relationships with in vivo data. Until sufficient validation is performed, it is not recommended that these data be used in ranking systems.

3) Varying degrees of technical sophistication may be expressed, depending on the depth of evaluation necessary in ranking/scoring procedures. Chronic toxicity, carcinogenicity, and acute toxicity scoring are active processes that depend on the current availability of data. Values used for any scoring procedure will need to reflect changing and improving data. The following types of updating should be considered for human health effects scoring.

   Error correction
   Study selection for chronic toxicity may often be based on secondary references to conserve staff resources in this screening exercise. A more detailed evaluation of primary sources for other internal programs could change the conclusion reached based on secondary sources. Similarly, if a regulatory agency should take a position on the quality or acceptability of a study used, the data could require review.

New data

As testing of chemicals continues through various programs, new infomation may become available, from industry, academia, or government, which would change a chemical's evaluation. More detailed evaluation of background information on a chemical could turn up data not previously cited in published, especially secondary references.

New regulatory action

Establishment of new toxicity values, revision of old values, changes in classification of carcinogens, or new classification of chemicals would change the evaluations included in this scoring procedure. Similarly, changes in evaluation techniques by regulatory agencies could require reevaluation of procedures used in this scoring system.

4) The utility of any scoring system is dependent on the data available to support the evaluation. Ready access to information on key components would support the application of screens by the broadest possible user base. The evaluation and decisions on health data should consistently be made to lead to selection of appropriate acute toxicity values and chronic NOAELs and development of weighting or calculation of potencies from carcinogenicity data. While general databases such as TOXLINE (National Library of Medicine [NLM] 1986) and HSDB compile toxicity studies, there is a clear need to develop a data source that would contain appropriately evaluated data for the components required for health effects screening. Such a database would include the acute toxicity values considered most representative for the chemical; the NOEL, NOAEL, or LOAEL considered most representative of the effects observed for the appropriate subcategories such as neurotoxicity, reproductive or developmental toxicity, immunotoxicity, organ system toxicity, etc.; and the data supporting the weighting of cancer data and ED10 calculations. The values included in the database should be appropriately peer reviewed and represent consensus evaluations of potential user communities. To a certain extent, the USEPA's IRIS database contains NOAEL and LOAEL information and potency slopes on chemicals reviewed for RfD and cancer risk development. The EU's regulatory International Uniform Chemical Information Database (IUCLID) will also contain some data evaluations and NOAEL and LOAEL values. Expansion of these systems or development of a system supporting retrieval of data critical to screening methods should be supported.

Chapter 4

Ecological Effects

Richard A. Kimerle, chapter editor
Lawrence W. Barnthouse, Richard P. Brown, Bernard Conilh de Beyssac,
Michael Gilbertson, Kathy Monk, Heinz-Jochen Poremski, Richard E. Purdy,
Kevin H. Reinert, Rosalind M. Rolland, Maurice G. Zeeman

The Ecological Effects Workgroup of the Society of Environmental Toxicology and Chemistry (SETAC) Chemical Ranking and Scoring (CRS) Workshop arrived at a general consensus on a number of the important issues for scoring and ranking chemicals for potential ecological effects. The workgroup agreed with the conclusion reached in the plenary workshop discussions that they should not prescribe "another" specific procedure for scoring and ranking chemicals for ecological effects. Instead, the technical foundation should be developed to provide guidance in evaluating existing procedures or in developing a new procedure to meet a specific goal not addressed by a current procedure. It was further recognized that the purposes of conducting CRS vary according to a user's program goals and needs. This suggests that various kinds of data are likely to be used and that the degree of appropriate technical sophistication will vary depending on the goals of the chemical scoring exercise. A multilevel, staged, or tiered approach was thought to be the most appropriate way to address the diversity of user needs. However, there is no reason to assume that the tiers would necessarily be implemented in sequential manner. In addition, the availability of data, or more likely lack thereof, will in many instances dictate which level or tier of technical sophistication and scientific rigor can be used.

It would be an ideal situation if ecological effects scoring were always risk-based. That is, data on exposure and ecological effects would be used to calculate a risk quotient (RQ) (effects concentration over exposure concentration), and then a score would be assigned to the RQ. However, this has not been done in existing scoring procedures, and thus the CRS workshop offered a very real opportunity to add this most significant dimension to scoring and ranking chemicals for potential ecological effects.

The overall intent of this chapter is to provide technical guidance in using existing and readily available data in several tiers from the simplest, where essentially no data are used, to a more scientifically defensible and rigorous risk-based tier that utilizes not just "hazard" or effects data but integrates exposure and effects data to arrive at an expression of risk.

Some of the specific purposes of this chapter are to

1) review the state-of-the-science for scoring potential ecological effects of chemicals while identifying opportunities to advance the science;

2) identify those ecological components or endpoints judged important enough to be included in the scientific foundation of chemical scoring to ecological effects;

3) suggest various tiers of effort and complexity (prescreening/flagging, screening, and risk-based) in scoring and ranking that can be useful in addressing the various needs of users;

4) identify some of the technical issues that influence the quality and usefulness of an ecological scoring procedure (data availability, data quality, data scoring alternatives; how to use quantitative structure-activity relationship (QSAR) data for early tier risk-based scoring); and

5) identify some of the research needed to advance the science of CRS.

State of the Science

Numerous scoring procedures have been developed to evaluate chemicals for potential adverse ecological effects. All are quite different with regard to the use of ecological data, goals, and purposes. For instance, the Informal working group on Priority Setting (IPS) scores and ranks chemicals on the basis of their potential danger to the environment based on a simple exposure-effect model (Emans 1993). The UCSS (USEPA 1993a) takes a different approach in which a set of chemicals and technologies are ranked and scored to assist in determining which substances may substitute for each other for a particular use. The reader is referred to the report by Davis et al. (1994) where many different approaches were reviewed.

Purposes of scoring for potential ecological effects

There are many different purposes and rationales for wanting to score and rank chemicals for potential ecological effects, resulting in a number of very different scoring procedures. Some of the purposes for which scoring and ranking procedures have been implemented are the following:

- screening chemicals for potential ecological effects;
- ranking numerous chemicals to focus attention on those that are most hazardous;
- regulatory decisions to restrict, label, ban, or set a standard, reducing a "set" of chemicals to a "manageable size" relative to the amount of resources available (time, personnel, money, effort);
- making internal business decisions for setting priorities, allocating limited resources, monitoring, judging need for more intensive testing or data collection, guiding business decisions (production, manufacturing, health, safety, design),

evaluating the need for specialized testing (bioaccumulation, endocrine disruption, teratology) and for remediation, pollution prevention, or restoration efforts;

- judging the need for more sophistication and complexity in an assessment;
- providing guidance to alternative chemical processes and products; and
- providing tiered priority lists for guiding mandatory or voluntary emissions reporting and emissions reduction efforts.

Basis of existing scoring procedures

Almost none of the existing chemical scoring procedures rely upon a risk-based approach for ecological effects (i.e., one that integrates the components of exposure potential with ecological effects data), depending instead upon toxicity, fate, or exposure data alone. This provides decision-makers with results that may not be founded in the best science available. Just because a chemical is inherently more toxic and achieves higher scores does not necessarily mean it has greater potential to cause adverse ecological effects. This deficiency in many of the published procedures was viewed as an opportunity to advance the science. However, it was also realized that many of these procedures have been designed as screening procedures only and perhaps do not warrant greater technical sophistication.

Traditional ecological endpoints

The ecological endpoints that have been most often used in scoring are related to the characteristics that are valued as ecologically relevant, have a substantial database, and have been relied upon in routine ecological testing and program management. The availability of quality data in the published open literature is one of the important features desirable to developing a quality scoring procedure. The characteristics or assessment endpoints most valued are toxicity, persistence, and bioaccumulation. Substances that strongly express these characteristics are referred to as the persistent, bioaccumulative, and highly toxic (PBT) chemicals. The parameters most often scored for the above 3 characteristics are acute lethal concentration to 50% of a test population (LC50), half-life in an environmental compartment, and bioconcentration factor (BCF), either estimated by an octanol–water partition coefficient (Kow) or measured in a bioconcentration uptake study.

The aquatic environment has been favored over the terrestrial environment because the most methods for testing chemicals for potential ecological effects have been performed with aquatic species. However, there has been a recent increased interest in wildlife bird and mammal toxicology testing for risk assessment purposes. For the aquatic environment, chemicals most often have been tested using acute toxicity assays on fish and on invertebrates such as *Daphnia magna*. Freshwater data are more prevalent than marine data. Terrestrial effects data are most often represented by rat acute oral data, with some data available for birds and other wildlife species.

The assessment endpoints of persistence and bioaccumulation are not strictly ecological parameters; they are more physical–chemical in nature and have a more direct influence on exposure than on biological effects. They are, however, viewed as being critically important to procedures for scoring ecological effects of chemicals. The reader is referred to Chapter 2, "Measures of Exposure," for additional details on the best method for establishing exposure scoring parameters. This chapter on ecological effects uses the exposure expressions of fate and persistence of chemicals as important components of ecological effects scoring.

Measured and QSAR data for scoring

There has been a great dependence on using measured data in many of the existing scoring procedures, especially for acute toxicity data. The science of scoring chemicals for potential ecological effects would probably be more advanced if more extensive databases were available. One problem with many of the existing CRS procedures is the way in which missing data are addressed. Some procedures simply cannot be performed on many chemicals because there are no alternatives for missing essential data. Some procedures "reward" missing data by defaulting the score to a low numeric value that offers no penalty and thus no incentive to obtain the data. Other procedures fill data gaps with estimates by using accepted QSAR procedures. In general, exposure estimates of persistence and bioaccumulation have relied more heavily on QSAR than on toxicity.

The development, validation, and availability of QSAR methods have provided increasingly powerful tools to estimate toxicity, degradation, and bioconcentration potential. Use of QSAR seems to be most prevalent and apparently accepted in procedures designed for screening purposes. Quantitative structure-activity relationship applications are able to provide some very useful, practical, and relevant estimates of toxic effects concentrations, both acute and chronic, and fate estimates when little or no "real" data are readily available (Clements et al. 1993; Nabholz et al. 1993; Zeeman et al. 1993, Zeeman 1995; Zeeman, Auer et al. 1995). Greater acceptance and better understanding of QSAR data for CRS are important challenges for the near future.

Characterizing Ecological Effects for CRS

A number of ecological effects components should be considered for inclusion in CRS procedures. The aim of this chapter is to provide a technical framework that can be used as guidance for characterizing these effects. Details provided in this chapter offer examples of how a technical scoring issue might be addressed. Users are encouraged to stay within the guidance while adapting the approach to their specific needs.

The important ecosystem criteria or assessment endpoints of interest here represent the earth's ecosystems and their structural and functional components. The aquatic and terrestrial environments were viewed as equally important in scoring procedures for assessing potential adverse ecological effects of chemicals. It is generally desirable to include representative or surrogate species from the trophic levels of primary producers (algae and higher plants), primary consumers and prey species (invertebrates such as daphnids and earthworms, avian species), and predators (fish, eagles, mammals) in a comprehensive scoring procedure. The vast majority of methods development for ecological effects testing has occurred for aquatic invertebrate and fish species. The rigor of scoring procedures would be enhanced if more data were available for aquatic and terrestrial plants, reptiles, amphibians, birds, and wildlife mammals.

Standardized laboratory toxicity test methods are available for a variety of aquatic and terrestrial species. The relatively small number of species in current test guidelines have usually been chosen to be representative surrogates for similar organisms in that grouping. For example, the rainbow trout and fathead minnow may serve to represent the thousands of freshwater fish species found in cold and warm freshwater environments, respectively. An important factor to remember is that the species that are able to be maintained in the laboratory may not adequately represent the most sensitive species found in the wild.

The most typical and important ecological characteristics that can be readily measured (i.e., endpoints) are survival, growth and development, and reproduction of the component species in ecosystems. The most commonly measured and available ecological endpoints are acute adverse effects, including

- lethal dose to 50% of a test population (LD50) for terrestrial species;
- LC50 for aquatic species;
- effective concentration to 50% of a test population (EC50) for various, sometimes difficult to define, endpoints for invertebrates; and
- EC50 for growth, total mass, or photosynthesis rate inhibition in higher plants.

Chronic data on growth and reproductive effect levels in long-term toxicity tests are not as frequently available as acute data and often must be estimated for aquatic species. These include

- lowest-observed-adverse-effect level (LOAEL),
- no-observed-adverse-effect level (NOAEL), and
- maximum allowable toxicant concentration (MATC).

Procedures for estimating chronic effects from acute data are presented in the "Data Issues" section.

The valid and available chemical toxicity test data for the aquatic environment typically consist of acute toxicity to freshwater fish (96-h LC50) and daphnids (48-h EC50). For example, the Duluth fathead minnow acute toxicity database (Brooke et al. 1984; Geiger et al. 1985, 1986, 1988, 1990) represents over 750 96-h LC50 tests on 651 specific organic chemicals in 24 chemical classes.

The aquatic toxicity test data that were assessed consisted of 920 effective test results for fish, daphnids, or algae on 462 chemicals. For these 462 chemicals, there were 414 fish 96-h LC50s, 307 daphnid 48-h LC50s, 145 green algal 96-h EC50s, 8 fish chronic values (MATCs), 14 daphnid MATCs, and 32 algal chronic values (Zeeman 1995).

Structure of Ecological Effects Scoring

It was recognized that with the multitude of purposes for scoring programs and the variations in quality and availability of required data, a need existed to provide the technical foundation for ecological effects scoring in tiers. The tiers that were identified, representing differing levels of complexity, utility, and data requirements were 1) hazard-based prescreening or flagging, 2) screening, and 3) risk-based scoring and ranking for potential ecological effects. Although these are presented as tiers, they are not necessarily intended to be used sequentially. Instead, each is considered a useful approach to meeting the intended purpose of the scoring activity. There is a tiered, sequential aspect to the 3 procedures, in that the data requirements and technical sophistication generally increase from the prescreen/flagging to the screening to the risk-based scoring procedure. Although the risk-based approach may be thought of as more data-intensive with requirements for both exposure and effects data, depending on the goals or purpose of the CRS, QSAR estimates can be used in lieu of missing data to conduct a useful ecological effects scoring activity. In general, if measured data are available, they should replace the QSAR data.

Prescreening and flagging chemicals for potential ecological effects

Prior to selecting the chemicals to be included in a formal first-level scoring exercise, it may be useful to perform a prescreen to select a subset of "substances of concern" to be reviewed further. This prescreening step will define the scope of the process (e.g., regional/global; organic/inorganic; single chemical, mixtures, or clusters; and minimum levels for toxicity, persistence, and bioaccumulation) and specify fundamental limitations (e.g., the minimum dataset required and acceptable data sources). The prescreening step should be simple and clear, requiring only limited data and very limited expert judgment (mainly a "mechanical" process).

This prescreening step can be contrasted to a final screening and scoring procedure, which may have the characteristics of
- requiring specific expert judgment,
- being consensus driven,
- being data intensive, and
- varying on a case-by-case basis.

Numerous examples can be given to illustrate the usefulness of a prescreen. Chemicals could be excluded from consideration when there is simply no likelihood for exposure to take place. For example, a chemical that is an intermediate in a chemical process and does not leave a reaction vessel could be a candidate for exclusion. Conversely, a prescreen may identify a chemical already known to be of concern based on monitoring data or its relationship to a chemical with known adverse environmental properties. For example, most highly chlorinated persistent chemicals could be handled as a class, especially if they were known to be continually loaded into the environment. Input to the prescreening should be at least conservative enough to include marginally important chemicals in the prescreening process. Candidate chemicals can move to a higher tier when prescreening results justify doing so. It is important that the prescreening stage in ecological scoring be conservative because traditional environmental risk assessment may not include all potentially adverse effects.

Traditional chemical screening methods for new or existing chemicals are primarily dependent upon controlled experimental models for toxicity testing and upon the use of theoretical modeling mechanisms for determining environmental fate. These fate models only provide estimates of environmental exposures and cannot accurately predict all of the potential biological effects of chemicals for the myriad species in a complex ecosystem. Therefore, if a chemical scoring system is based upon these methods, it risks neglecting chemicals that are capable of causing significant biological effects under actual environmental conditions.

Experimental toxicity testing can address only a limited number of endpoints in a limited number of species. It is practically impossible to include all potentially exposed organisms from an ecosystem in the testing paradigm. Thus, the potential biological impact of a chemical on an environmentally exposed, sensitive species could be overlooked by extrapolating between species. Furthermore, chemicals are tested on an individual basis, and the environmental mixing of chemicals with possible additive, synergistic, or antagonistic effects is not considered. Theoretical environmental loading calculations typically do not include variables such as contributions from atmospheric transportation and deposition or other additional inputs of chemicals (e.g., from bordering countries). Nonpersistent, non-bioaccumulative chemicals are often thought to present less of an environmental threat than PBT chemicals; however, if they are continually released, a constant level of exposure to organisms will be maintained, posing a unique hazard potential. Similarly, if they are continually released at a loading rate that exceeds their degradation or assimilation rate, exposure levels may even increase over time.

Finally, a limited number of biological endpoints are measured during toxicity testing. Current systems do not address the more subtle biological endpoints of long-term, low-level chemical exposures that are more typical in the environment. For example, wildlife epidemiological studies have raised concern about untested transgenerational and endocrine-disrupting effects resulting from environmental exposure to certain synthetic chemicals, and although these relationships are not clear-cut, damage of that nature to wildlife populations has been documented.

For all of the above reasons, it is recommended that epidemiological data on ecological hazards of synthetic chemicals be acknowledged early in the chemical scoring process (e.g., by flagging).

Wildlife epidemiology/ecotoxicology field studies take place in an uncontrolled and complex environment. Investigators have developed a weight-of-evidence approach to establish causal relationships between environmental chemical exposures and observed biological effects in a wildlife population, which may be a useful input to a CRS prescreening stage. This approach is based upon 6 criteria to establish the cause-and-effect relationship between a chemical exposure and an observed biological effect in field studies. Of necessity, this approach is applicable only to chemicals already present in the environment. These weight-of-evidence criteria are listed below.

- Time order: Did the exposure to the putative chemical agent precede manifestation of the observed biological effect?
- Specificity: Does the putative chemical agent lead only to the effect, and does only the putative agent lead to the effect?
- Strength of association: Do the distributions of the incidence of the effect and of the putative chemical agent co-vary?
- Consistency on replication: Have other researchers, using other research designs in other locations and at other times on other species, found the same relationship?
- Coherence: Do the facts cohere to existing biological theory, and are there plausible routes of exposure?
- Performance on prediction: Has the cause-and-effect relationship predicted new phenomena that logically follow from the observations?

Chemicals that meet the weight-of-evidence criteria could be flagged to indicate a preexisting association with detrimental biological effects in the ecosystem and, thus, identify a special priority for concern.

It can be a valuable exercise to look for flags that raise some level of concern when reviewing a chemical's database or its life-cycle portfolio. Integrating these flags into a CRS system is recommended for the following reasons:

1) There is a need to keep track of significant information and drivers that are responsible for the interim or final score. Important drivers can include, e.g., high persistence or bioaccumulation potential.

2) There is a need to integrate nonconventional but relevant assessment endpoints into the system, without unbalancing the more conventional use of practical considerations.

Integrating nonconventional ecological assessment endpoints (e.g., reduction of biodiversity, loss of ecosystem functions) without clarifying what is currently practical may result in unrealistic expectations. However, presenting only conventional ecological assessment endpoints will reduce the likelihood of scientific advances.

When new ecological assessment endpoints are integrated, the appropriate degree of extrapolation depends upon the acceptable degree of uncertainty. Therefore, new ecological assessment endpoints may be more easily integrated into a system where uncertainty is explicitly characterized and accounted for in subsequent decision-making.

Examples of possible new ecological assessment endpoints and explicit expressions of environmental values to be protected that could be considered in a prescreen (provided, of course, that data are or become available) include these:
* biodiversity assessment;
* endocrinological effects;
* developmental effects;
* long-term cumulative effects;
* immunological effects;
* transgeneration effects;
* marine ecosystem effects; and
* documented synergistic, antagonistic, or additive effects.

Biodiversity assessment endpoints that could be part of a prescreen should consider ecosystem diversity, species diversity, and genetic diversity. Ecosystem diversity issues include the following:
* endangered ecosystems (e.g., tall grass prairie);
* ecologically important or sensitive ecosystems (e.g., wetlands);
* unique ecosystems (e.g., hot springs); and
* protected ecosystems (e.g., parks, wetlands designated to be of international importance [Ramsar Convention 1976], sanctuaries, wildlife areas, and reserves).

Species diversity issues include the following:
* nationally designated species (e.g., endangered species, threatened, and vulnerable species);
* endemic species;
* keystone or ecologically important species;
* economically important species (e.g., crops and livestock species, fisheries species, forestry species);
* internationally protected species (e.g., migratory birds, polar bears, porcupine caribou herd); and
* other species of importance to the public.

Genetic diversity issues include these:

- genetic diversity important for species adaptability (endangered species, wild plants, other valued species);
- genetic material of value for animal or plant breeding; and
- other genetic material of commercial importance for biotechnology.

Developing biodiversity measurement endpoints requires special consideration of the following:

- When it is not possible to measure assessment endpoints directly, there will be a need for extrapolation guidelines (e.g., the taxonomic hierarchy approach).
- Because of the special value of endangered species, the selection of measurement endpoints for them may be more similar to approaches for assessing risks to humans (where every individual matters).
- Where toxicity data are available for a valued species, the lethal dose to 10% or 1% of a test population (LD10 or LD1) may be more a appropriate measurement endpoint than LD50. It must be recognized, however, that these types of data are often unavailable, whereas LC50, EC50, and IC50 (inhibitory concentration to 50% of a test population) data are quite common.

First tier scoring

The first tier (or Tier 1) procedure to score chemicals should use those endpoints for which data are generally available or for which estimates can be made. The endpoints should also be relevant to the specific goals or purpose of the prioritizing or ranking. At a minimum, 3 endpoints are recommended: persistence, bioaccumulation, and toxicity. These endpoints are used in the examples and discussion below. The actual choice of endpoints for any particular use and the general availability of data for various endpoints are discussed below.

In Tier 1, the endpoints may be treated in 2 ways: 1) as a threshold, or trigger, where a chemical exceeding the trigger for any 3 of the 4 endpoints would be selected or 2) by a scoring and ranking procedure where the 3 endpoints are combined and the chemicals are scored and/or ranked. The purposes of Tier 1 might be to prioritize chemicals, to identify chemicals for additional review, or to identify needs for additional data. Use of Tier 1 is most appropriate when the number of chemicals to be reviewed is large compared to the resources available and/or the data available for the initial review are very limited. The product of a Tier 1 CRS will be, in the case of 1) above, 2 groups of chemicals that either have been selected for some purpose or excluded from consideration. In the case of 2) above, the product will be an array of the chemicals that have been assigned a relative score.

Combining available PBT data

For each of the 3 endpoints suggested in Tier 1, the available information could be condensed to a single measurement. Selection of a single-number toxicity value may be facilitated by considering the following:

- worst-case single toxicity value within trophic levels or among trophic levels,
- geometric mean toxicity value within trophic levels or among trophic levels,
- percentile toxicity value within trophic levels or among trophic levels, or
- combination of the above procedures.

Selecting toxicity, persistence, and bioaccumulation data should also include considerations for selecting the highest quality data. In general, the use of the worst-case value guards against false negatives, i.e., not selecting a chemical for further review when it should be included. It is also thought to address the variation in species sensitivity in the wild compared to the few species tested. The use of this method would be most appropriate in Tier 1 when the object is to ensure that all chemicals that should be selected for review are selected. It is important when using the worst-case value that the test result is not an anomaly, i.e., it is based on a quality study or a reliable estimation method. A geometric mean makes use of all of the available information while weighing the lowest values more heavily. In general, the use of the geometric mean is appropriate when the purpose is to make a comparative analysis rather than a screening analysis.

Conversion to or use of chronic data

Use of chronic data in Tier 1 may be more attractive than acute data for many purposes but is not necessary, nor are such data frequently available. As the "Data Issues in Ecological Effects" section indicates, there are methods to estimate chronic values based on acute data. This may be addressed by one of the following methods:

- Use the acute value directly with no conversion or modification. If no actual chronic data are available or if the conversion is done by the use of the same factor for every chemical, there is no reason to convert acute values to chronic values for ranking purposes.
- Use a measured acute-to-chronic ratio. If these ratios are different for different chemicals, then this process adds additional information useful in making distinctions for ranking; it also then allows the inclusion of whatever measured chronic data are available. This is particularly useful in dealing with classes of chemicals.
- Divide by a factor of 10 to approximate a no-observed-effect concentration (NOEC). If the Tier 1 method went beyond the 3 most basic endpoints included here, e.g., if it included fate parameters that addressed specific compartments or more directly addressed actual exposure, then the toxicity measure might also be adjusted to more closely approximate a level having some actual interpretation in the environment. If this were done in a meaningful way, then the resulting final rank might have an interpretation more easily related to recognized categories of concern in the environment.

- Divide by a factor of 100 to approximate a concentration level "of concern" (see paragraph above).

Use of thresholds or triggers

In a threshold/trigger system, trigger or threshold values are specified for each endpoint. Exceeding the trigger for any of the 3 endpoints prompts selection for further review. This method is illustrated below. If any of the values indicates a level of concern greater than that for the trigger, then the chemical is selected for the next action step, which could be further data gathering, evaluating the chemical to a category of greater concern, or eliminating the chemical from consideration in favor of a lower scoring chemical (e.g., when creating a list of preferred chemicals).

Triggers could be set to select only those chemicals that may actually be of concern in the environment. However, choosing to do so depends on the goals or purpose of the particular project. For example, resources may be limited and further evaluation can take place on only a given number of chemicals. Clearly, the trigger values that are set will determine how many chemicals are selected from Tier 1. If resources dictate that only a certain number of chemicals may be addressed for further action, the triggers may have to be revised to "catch" fewer chemicals.

The typical output of this process is a listing of 2 categories of chemicals: a group of selected chemicals and a group of unselected chemicals. However, it is very important that the chemicals be flagged (e.g., P, T, and/or B) to indicate on what basis they were selected. This is important in explaining the results of the screen. It may also be useful if it is necessary to rank the chemicals selected in the screen. For example, chemicals selected for all 3 endpoints may be put into the highest priority category; chemicals with a P and T might be in a separate category; and those chemicals that triggered only one endpoint may also form other categories, e.g., the Accelerated Reduction/Elimination of Toxics (ARET) System (Environment Canada and OMOEE 1994) and Ontario's "Candidate Substances for Bans, Phase-outs or Reductions" selection protocol (Socha et al. 1992), again depending on the purposes of the exercise.

A major limitation of this type of screening is that it does not produce a single specific score. Therefore, it may be difficult to combine the results with other measures such as production or release volume. However, this may be overcome if, for example, the chemicals are arranged into categories as described above and ranking scores are assigned to these groups as illustrated in Table 4-1.

Table 4-1 Single scores reflecting ecological effects thresholds or triggers

Flags	Measurement scale
T,P,B	5
T,P	4
T,B	3
P,B	3
T	2
P	2
B	2
no flags	1

Ordering/scoring screening model

In the ordering/scoring model, a measurement scale is developed for each of the endpoints. For each chemical, the scores on each of the scales are combined to give an overall score for the ecological effects component. Table 4-2 offers a purely arbitrary example that will be used to illustrate certain principles.

Table 4-2 Scores for ecological effects

Measurement scale	Acute toxicity (mg/L)	Persistence (half-life, d)	BCF
5	< 0.01	> 100	> 5
4	0.01 to 0.1	50 to 100	4 to 5
3	0.1 to 1.0	10 to 50	3 to 4
2	1.0 to 10.0	2 to 10	2 to 3
1	> 10 to 100	0.5 to 2	1 to 2
0	> 100	< 0.5	< 1

Many measurement scales in the ecological effects area have been developed based on more or less arbitrary cutoff points or categorizations (e.g., log scales, percentile cutoffs based on available data). Although this may be necessary in many cases, the aim should be to develop categories that reflect meaningful distinctions or that, when combined with the other available endpoints, create distinctions that are ecologically meaningful for ranking chemicals. In general, the more arbitrary the original measurement scales, the more arbitrary the final scores will be.

For example, looking at the persistence endpoint in the example above (Table 4-2), the intervals defined on the scale may not be meaningful if the primary compartment of concern is aquatic organisms. Because many aquatic invertebrate life cycles are measured in days, the persistence scale would need to be revised so that the intervals begin at a much shorter time frame and the defined categories have much smaller time intervals.

Once measurement scales have been constructed, endpoints may be aggregated in a variety of ways. In selecting and evaluating an aggregation method, it is important to examine the results of the method. The final scores or rankings should make realistic distinctions and should not make distinctions that are unwarranted.

One useful way to evaluate score aggregation is to carefully examine the end results by looking at all of the ways in which chemicals can be assigned a particular final score and by determining if these are equivalent. For example, if we were to combine P and T by adding the scores for P and T given in Table 4-3, the final aggregate scores for PT would range from 1 to 10. There would then be five ways to obtain a score of "6" for PT as shown in Table 4-3:

Table 4-3 Aggregate scores for persistence and toxicity

Toxicity (mg/L)	Toxicity score	Persistence (half-life, d)	Persistence score	P + T score
< 0.01	5	< 2	1	6
0.01 to 0.1	4	2 to 10	2	6
0.1 to1.0	3	10 to 50	3	6
1.0 to10	2	50 to 100	4	6
>10	1	> 100	5	6

A determination can then be made whether these combinations are equivalent, i.e., that chemicals with the same score are of equal concern for whatever purpose the scoring system is to be used. A similar exercise can be conducted for the other combinations that lead to equivalent scores (e.g., the five ways to get a "5," the four ways to get a "7," etc.). If any equivalencies are not plausible, then it may be necessary and justifiable to change the aggregation method or reorganize the final scale (e.g., into fewer categories). The results should be consistent with professional judgment.

Risk-based scoring

In this approach, the intent is to reflect the steps that would be taken in conducting a quantitative risk assessment (QRA), to maximize transparency, and to minimize the influence of artifacts introduced by scoring procedures. These artifacts are inevitable because different algorithms (addition, multiplication, etc.) for assigning and aggregating scores can be expected to produce different rankings for the scored chemicals. In addition, a risk-based approach is desirable for many scoring applications because 1) it most closely parallels the regulatory risk assessments that might ultimately be performed for chemicals scored as "potentially hazardous" or identified as "potentially safe" substitutes for existing chemicals, and 2) it facilitates the use of the methodology in product life-cycle assessments or pollution prevention programs where comparative risk assessments are used to evaluate alternative products or processes. Little or no more information is required for risk-based scoring than is already required in many existing CRS systems.

As a first step in the risk-based scoring approach, the equilibrium environmental partitioning of each chemical is estimated using a simple environmental fate model such as "unit world" fugacity models (e.g., Mackay 1991; Cowan et al. 1995). The Level I fugacity model determines the fraction of chemical partitioned into various environmental compartments (e.g., air, water, and sediment, soil, suspended matter, and biota). Chapter 2 discusses the use of fugacity-type models to estimate environmental concentrations in more detail.

For aquatic biota in the water column or sediment, an RQ can be directly calculated from an NOEC and an exposure concentration.

For water:

$$RQ = \frac{\text{Water Concentration (mg/L)}}{\text{Chronic NOEC (mg/L)}}$$

Or for sediment:

$$RQ = \frac{\text{Sediment Concentration (mg/kg)}}{\text{Chronic NOEC (mg/kg)}}$$

Risk quotients can be converted to risk scores according to any of the methods described above under Tier 1. For example, the conversions in Table 4-4 could be used.

Table 4-4 Assigning scores to risk quotients

	RQ			
< 0.1	0.1 to 1	1 to 10	10 to 100	> 100
Score 0	1	2	3	4

A significant disadvantage of this scoring method is that the information contained in the quotients is not retained. Risk quotients calculated using the approach described in this section are "interval-scaled" relative risk estimates. This means that the magnitude of the difference in RQs between 2 chemicals is an estimate of their relative risk. A similar scoring system that retains interval scaling could use the equation

$$\text{Score} = \log_{10}(RQ + 1) \tag{4-1}.$$

If RQs are calculated for multiple media or endpoints, then an aggregation step may be required to provide a single ecological risk score. Aggregation can be accomplished according to any one of the numerous approaches described in this chapter or in Chapters 1 and 3.

The risk-based scoring procedure described above deals directly with aquatic biota only. The principal reason for this limitation is that, whereas aquatic systems have been a major subject for ecotoxicological research and risk assessment for decades, terrestrial systems have received significant attention only recently. Non-aquatic ecological receptors are also important to consider in CRS. For terrestrial biota, such as wildlife, additional assumptions would be necessary to calculate RQ because air, water, and soil concentrations alone are insufficient to estimate wildlife exposures. The steps that would be required to estimate RQs for terrestrial biota are discussed below.

Piscivorous birds can be relatively easily accommodated in the risk-based scoring procedure discussed above. Many studies have documented high exposure of these birds to bioaccumulating contaminants; impacts on populations in the Great Lakes region and elsewhere have been demonstrated. Concentrations of contaminants (mg/kg) in fish can be obtained from simple partitioning models, either as a direct model output or by applying a BCF to a sediment or water-column concentration estimate. Estimation of a dose rate to a fish-eating bird (mg/day) requires knowledge of consumption rates (kg/day) for typical piscivorous birds. We know of no current scoring or screening models that include this information, but it is readily available from the avian literature and from the USEPA's Wildlife Exposure Factors Handbook (USEPA 1993b).

Avian toxicity tests are not routinely performed for chemicals other than pesticides. However, as a first approximation, mammalian (e.g., rodent) data may be used. Mammalian data must be used with caution, however, because differences in mammalian versus avian physiology (especially reproductive physiology) may produce wide divergences in sensitivity for some types of chemicals. A prescreening flag for chemicals whose structure indicates a possibility for such differences would be extremely useful. Once an NOAEL has been established, an RQ can be calculated and scored according to any of the procedures described above.

Marine systems are not addressed directly in any of the scoring procedures described in this report. There are sound scientific reasons to believe that, at least as a first approximation, freshwater systems can serve as a surrogate. Partitioning of most organic contaminants between air, water, and sediment is not strongly affected by salinity, and comparative toxicity studies have demonstrated that the sensitivity of different biota to contaminants is more strongly correlated with taxonomic affinity than with freshwater versus saltwater habitat. Marine mammals, however, represent a special case. These animals have often been found to accumulate high concentrations of many contaminants. It appears feasible to use the same dose estimation methods for marine mammals as for piscivorous birds. Mammalian toxicity data would be clearly as appropriate for estimating toxicity of chemicals to marine mammals as for estimating toxicity to humans. Differences in availability due to saltwater versus freshwater chemistry may be important for some types of contaminants; these may be predictable from chemical structure.

Terrestrial ecosystems are not dealt with directly in this book. Terrestrial animals can be exposed to contaminants through the same pathways as humans can be exposed (e.g., inhalation, water contact, drinking water, food, soil contact, and direct soil consumption). Simple partitioning models do not explicitly simulate these pathways. A variety of site-specific models for quantifying the movement of contaminants from soil and water to plants and animals exists. These models require species-specific consumption estimates and site-specific environmental data and are not directly suitable for chemical scoring. Suitably generic models could undoubtedly be developed; however, it may be acceptable for comparative scoring or ranking purposes to use aquatic systems as a surrogate. Even when contaminants are deposited on land, water and sediment are often the ultimate sinks, as has been the case with polychlorinated biphenyls (PCBs) and dichlorodiphenyl trichloroethane (DDT) deposited in the Great Lakes Basin and mercury deposited in the Arctic. One significant potential disadvantage of using aquatic systems as a surrogate is the failure to assess impacts on terrestrial vegetation. Lack of information on effects of chemicals other than herbicides on plants is a common obstacle for all scoring systems. Currently there are few standardized test systems for plants and no reliable QSARs. It is, however, possible to use an understanding of plant physiology to develop flags for potential plant toxicity based on chemical structure, e.g., as in the USEPA Mid-continent Ecology Division (MED)/Montana State University's computerized QSAR system.

Off-the-shelf tools for risk-based scoring

There are software packages available that will predict the fate of chemicals and compare them to toxicity values. There is also software available to estimate all of the properties required by the fate and toxicity models.

For example, the Uniform System for the Evaluation of Substances (USES), developed in the Netherlands (Vermeire et al. 1994), is based on a steady-state Level III multi-media chemical fate model called SimpleBOX (van de Meent 1993). Cowan et al. (1995) describe this and other Mackay-type multi-media models. These models typically require input on amounts and modes of environmental release as well as the following chemical properties: log of the Kow (LogP); vapor pressure (Pv); molecular weight (MW); half-lives in water, air, and sediments; and LC50 and/or other toxicity measures. These values or surrogates can be calculated with software available from various sources. Syracuse Research Corporation has a software package, Estimation Programs Interface (EPI©) (SRC 1996), that will estimate all properties except LC50. LC50s can be obtained from Ecotoxicity of Industrial Chemicals Based on Structure-Activity Relationships (ECOSAR) (USEPA 1994b) or Assessment Tools for the Evaluation of Risk (ASTER) (Russom 1994). Other software packages are available for estimating these properties, but the aforementioned are of known utility for this purpose. The software could be linked as illustrated in Figure 4-1.

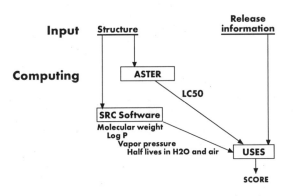

Figure 4-1 Linking software for risk-based scoring

Use of epidemiological data for validation or refinement

How well do chemical scoring systems predict the potential for adverse ecosystem impacts of a given chemical? A feedback mechanism that compares chemical screening prioritization with actual environmental fate and biological effects in an ecosystem could provide a method to assess the predictive ability of the scoring system in terms of ecosystem impacts. Also, field data on exposure and observed biological effects or lack of effects could provide input on the relative applicability and significance of the endpoints and species used in experimental studies of toxicity. This comparison would provide feedback information for future refinement and/or validation of experimental testing and modeling components (e.g., biological endpoints, species tested).

Data Issues in Ecological Effects Scoring

Use of quantitative structure-activity relationships

Valid aquatic or terrestrial toxicity test data often are not available for many industrial chemicals. When such test data are not available, it is increasingly common to make structure–activity relationship (SAR) and QSAR predictions. Structure-activity relationships and QSARs are available for many classes of discrete organic chemicals, and they can be used as additional sources of toxicity data. There are many published QSARs for aquatic effects. Most of these are for single classes or small sets of compounds, with a few unified systems that cover a broad spectrum of chemicals in a uniform manner. There are insufficient numbers of QSARs for effects on terrestrial organisms.

Most of the QSARs for aquatic organisms are for predicting acute lethality (LC50) values for fish. There are also some algal and invertebrate acute QSARs; there are fewer chronic QSARs available. For scoring, available standard QSARs or systems are probably best. The following are the 2 most popular and useful at this time.

1) ECOSAR (USEPA 1994b): This program was developed for use with personal computers and is distributed by USEPA's Office of Pollution Prevention and Toxics (OPPT). It is a compilation of QSARs from the literature and those developed internally by OPPT. The QSARs are for various chemical classes like esters, aliphatic alcohols, tertiary amines, polynuclear aromatics, etc. To obtain a prediction, a user chooses a chemical class based on the presence of certain functional groups. Then the MW and log Kow are entered by the user. For some chemicals, such as surfactants or polymers, the charge density (e.g., average number of carbons in the alkyl chain or percent amine nitrogen) must be known. The system provides an acute LC50 for fish, *Daphnia*, and chronic predictions for these and for algae if possible, although for many classes not all predictions can be made.

   The recent United States/European Union SAR/MPD study (OECD 1994; USEPA 1994d) has also demonstrated that USEPA's aquatic toxicity SAR/QSAR predictions were very often able to suitably estimate the Minimum Premarket Dataset (MPD) aquatic toxicity base-set test data being received by the EU. The use of SAR/QSAR for terrestrial organisms is also starting to be used (Zeeman, Fairbrother, Gorsuch 1995).

2) Assessment Tools for the Evaluation of Risk (ASTER) is a combination database and QSAR. It was developed by the USEPA MED in Duluth, Minnesota (Russom

1994). Availability is limited outside of USEPA. The system predicts fathead minnow LC50 as well as properties such as boiling point (BP), melting point, water solubility (S), Kow, and dissociation constant (pKa) from chemical structure. The predictions are based on Kow calculated by the system and a set of complex rules in the program for identifying the mechanism of toxicity. These rules identify the class to which a chemical belongs. The user only has to provide chemical structure in the Simplified Molecular Line Input System (SMILES) format (Weininger et al. 1986). The output includes the probable mechanism of action (e.g., polar narcosis, nonpolar narcosis, alkylation, and uncoupling). The system can also provide all of the best literature values for toxicity as the user directs.

In addition, the model described by Verhaar et al. (1992) has been included in various proposals by the Netherlands National Institute of Public Health and Environmental Protection (RIVM) and the Organization for Economic Cooperation and Development (OECD) as an approach for classifying and obtaining LC50 values for chemicals. This paper provides rules for classifying chemicals as nonpolar narcotics. The chemicals in this class can then have their LC50 values predicted from octanol–water partition coefficients. Other mechanisms of toxicity are given, and examples of such chemicals are listed in tables. However, no rules are given for classifying chemicals into broad classes. Work is underway to develop the appropriate rules. Fewer classes are proposed by this paper than the number ECOSAR uses, but they have the potential to be more universal. If and when such universal classes and QSARs are developed, we will be able to predict toxicity more accurately for most chemicals.

Tests methods and data quality

Testing on new chemicals will require the application of internationally harmonized test methods such as OECD (1993, 1994) Test Guidelines and the application of good laboratory practice (GLP) rules. This ensures sufficient data quality. All other data sources need to be examined with regard to their validity and plausibility. Information on the test reports, details of testing procedures, and a comparison by using QSARs of similar structures would help in performing this check on validity and plausibility.

Assessment factors and principles to derive NOECs

The currently practiced approaches on hazard assessment use the NOECs from test species such as fish, *Daphnia*, and algae, which represent the 3 main trophic levels of an aquatic ecosystem. When facing the complexity of a multispecies ecosystem and the interactions in a real-life environment, a number of uncertainties must be considered by using single-species laboratory data such as

- intra- and interlaboratory variation of toxicity data,
- intra- and interspecies variations,
- differently sensitive biological endpoints, and
- laboratory-to-field extrapolation.

This requires that a minimum confidence factor of 10 be applied to the NOEC of the most sensitive species in order to carry out an assessment. If there are fewer data available on different taxonomic groups, short-term exposure-related toxicity data are available; if less sensitive endpoints are investigated, these must be taken into account by applying additional modification factors describing the degree of uncertainty when establishing and using these data for further assessment. (The suggested use of a confidence factor is analogous to the use of modifying factors described in Chapter 3. It is important to keep transparent the use of any confidence or modifying factor in a CRS system.)

The following describes a widely accepted procedure used by the OECD and the EU to ascertain appropriate modification factors depending on the availability of different types of toxicity data. There may be specific and well-reasoned cases where the assessment factors could be varied as described in the explanatory notes (EU 1993; EC 1994).

Assessment factor of 1,000, when available data include

- at least 1 short-term LC50 or EC50 from each of 3 trophic levels (fish, *Daphnia*, algae).

  Note: This is a conservative and protective factor designed to ensure that substances with the potential to cause adverse effects are identified in the effects assessment. In some circumstances, it may be necessary to raise or lower the assessment factor depending on the evidence available. Such evidence could include that from structurally similar compounds, knowledge of the mode of action, availability of data from a wide selection of species covering additional taxonomic groups other than those represented by the base-set species, and/or availability of data from a variety of species covering the taxonomic groups of the base-set species across at least 3 trophic levels. (In such a case, the assessment factors may be lower only if these multiple data points are available for the most sensitive taxonomic group.) Variation from a factor of 1,000 should be fully supported by accompanying evidence. Under no circumstances should a factor lower than 100 be used in deriving a predicted no-effect concentration (PNEC) from short-term toxicity data.

Assessment factor of 100, when available data include
- at least 1 short-term LC50 or EC50 from each of 3 trophic levels (fish, *Daphnia*, algae) and
- 1 long-term NOEC (either fish or *Daphnia*).

  Note: This applies to a single long-term NOEC (fish or *Daphnia*) if the NOEC was generated for the taxa/trophic level showing the lowest LC50 or EC50 in the short-term tests. It applies also to the lower of 2 long-term NOECs covering 2 taxa/trophic levels when such NOECs have not been generated from that showing the lowest LC50 or EC50 of the short-term tests.

Assessment factor of 50, when available data include
- at least 1 short-term LC50 or EC50 from each of 3 trophic levels (fish, *Daphnia,* algae) and
- 2 long-term NOECs from species representing 2 trophic levels (fish and/or *Daphnia* and/or algae).

  Note: This applies to the lower of 2 NOECs covering 2 taxa/trophic levels when such NOECs have been generated covering the lowest LC50 or EC50 in the short-term tests. It also applies to the lowest of 3 NOECs covering 3 taxa/trophic levels when such NOECs have not been generated from that showing the lowest LC50 or EC50 in the short-term tests.

Assessment factor of 10, when available data include
- long-term NOECs from at least 3 species (normally fish, *Daphnia,* and algae) representing 3 trophic levels.

  Note: The PNEC should be calculated from the lowest available NOEC that is consistent with other data. Extrapolation to the ecosystem effects can be made with much greater confidence, and thus a reduction of the assessment factor of 10 is possible. This is only sufficient, however, if the species tested can be considered to represent one of the more sensitive groups, i.e., if data were available on at least 3 species across 3 trophic levels. It may sometimes be possible to determine with high probability that the most sensitive species has been examined, i.e., that further long-term NOEC from a different taxonomic group would not be lower than the data already available. In those circumstances, a factor of 10 applied to the lowest NOEC from only 2 species would also be appropriate, especially if the substance does not have a potential to bioaccumulate. If it is not possible to make this judgment, then an assessment factor of 50 should be applied to take into account any interspecies variation in sensitivity. A factor of 10 cannot be decreased on the basis of laboratory studies.

The USEPA Office of Toxic Substances (OTS) has also developed assessment factors to be used in setting concern levels or concern concentrations for new industrial chemicals (USEPA 1984b), summarized in Table 4-5. Zeeman and Gilford (1993) and Zeeman (1995) provide further information on USEPA's use of assessment factors.

Table 4-5 Assessment factors for setting concern concentrations

Available data	Assessment factor
Limited (e.g., one acute test or acute SAR/QSAR for chemical or analogue)	1,000
Base-set acute toxicity (e.g., algal, daphnid, and fish testing) on chemical or analogue	100
Chronic toxicity of chemical or analogue	10
Field test data	1

Ecological Effects Research Needs

Several potential research needs have been identified. Additionally, some issues were not included because they were too complex to be encompassed in a CRS scheme. The following issues were identified as requiring additional research before being considered for inclusion into a scoring framework.

1) Mode of action: Although under consideration as a flag or "alarm" requiring additional action for chemicals associated with specific modes of action, the rules for associating such modes of action with particular chemicals have been developed only to a limited extent. Additional effort needs to be given to determining which modes of action could be listed as potential problems.

2) Soil exposure: Although soil concentrations can be estimated by fugacity models (e.g., Mackay Level I and II), their association in a scientifically defensible manner with ecological endpoints of concern is unclear. Some effort was expended regarding conservative comparisons by setting the exposure (e.g., the amount of a chemical consumed by the terrestrial organisms) to mammalian and avian species equal to the estimated soil concentration. While this is acceptable for earthworms, it is an unreasonable worst-case assumption for other receptors. Unfortunately, earthworm data availability was considered limited and not readily usable as a terrestrial receptor in this general scoring framework. Of course, earthworm data could be used in a modified or refined scoring procedure for a particular purpose. Also, limited earthworm QSARs are available.

3) Plants: Aquatic plants are represented typically by algae. Higher level aquatic plant data typically are not available for most chemicals. Again, soil exposure concentrations can be estimated, but it is unclear whether to include terrestrial plants as receptors for soil contaminants. Only root exposure and uptake dependent on the characteristics of a chemical would be assessed. QSARs for estimating higher terrestrial plant toxicity are not generally available; it is recommended that they be developed. Additionally, many compounds may expose plants via the atmosphere. Relative concentrations in air could be output from the exposure model; however, this procedure is the subject of future Mackay model refinements that are currently in progress. These concentrations could be modified by generally available QSAR fate processes for compounds that partition into the atmosphere.

4) Causality; epidemiology: Consistent with the identified need to explore and define new or potentially problematic modes of action, we often find effects in the environment for which causality cannot be determined. A current example is endocrine disruption, for which the exact causes in the environment have not been adequately elucidated. Such an endpoint could be added to a refined or modified scoring procedure based on the purpose of the scoring, but how do we determine which additional, potentially unknown endpoints should be addressed? Investiga-

tion of ecological epidemiology procedures and potential endpoints is recommended.

5) Avian chronic toxicity: The current ecological effects element does not include this endpoint, either directly or indirectly, primarily due to lack of data (except for pesticides) or methods for estimation. Additionally, QSARs for deriving both acute and chronic avian toxicities from available data do not appear to have been formally developed.

6) Marine ecosystem receptors: Marine ecosystems were not formally included in the ecological effects element. The workgroup thought that estuarine marine fish and invertebrates were adequately represented by test results from freshwater fish and invertebrates. Usually the sensitivity between freshwater and marine species is similar except that solubility of compounds in salt water is lower, tending to drive the chemical into the organism to a higher but not significant extent. Marine mammals and birds have not been addressed by the scoring system examples given but could be considered if the purpose or use of the scoring system was directed toward estuarine or marine systems.

7) Technology transfer: Numerous QSAR programs can evaluate both physical–chemical fate properties and ecological effect endpoints. Unfortunately, the existence of these programs, the specifics surrounding their potential use, and the actual current uses of these systems are not widely known. Many research groups may be able to demonstrate specific and unique uses for these programs, which can greatly enhance the ability of scoring systems to appropriately score chemicals. Enhancing and disseminating the understanding and use of these very important data estimation programs is recommended.

8) Interspecies relevance: There is a need to determine the degree of relevance of animal and human health data to aquatic and other environmental receptors, and vice-versa.

Chapter 5

Other Chemical Characteristics

Allan A. Jensen, John D. Walker, chapter editors
Franz Fiala, Karim Ahmed, Mark Ralston, Robert Ross,
Fredrich Schmidt-Bleek, Duane Tolle

The purpose of this chapter is to 1) provide examples of other characteristics that have been less commonly used in existing chemical ranking and scoring (CRS) systems to date; 2) discuss how these characteristics could be added to existing systems or used in future CRS systems; and 3) suggest how a tiered approach could be used to integrate these with more often-used criteria.

State of the Science

Davis et al. (1994) identified several other substance characteristics used in existing CRS systems that could not be classified as human health effects, ecological effects, or measures of exposure. The most common of these characteristics are chemical properties relating to physical effects or physical hazards, such as

- ignitability/flammability,
- flashpoint (FP),
- boiling point (BP),
- oxidizing properties,
- reactivity (instability),
- explosivity, and
- corrosivity.

Other properties such as taste, odor, and appearance have been used in CRS, although much less frequently than those listed above. Examples of the use of these various other characteristics include the following:

- Systematic Data Collection and Handling for Priority Setting (Gjøs et al. 1989) assigns scores for physical properties based on a chemical's BP, FP, and explosivity.
- The Michigan Critical Materials Register (MCMR) (MDNR 1987) includes criteria for physical and chemical properties and aesthetics in evaluating chemicals. U.S. National Fire Prevention Association (NFPA) ratings (described in the section

titled "Ignitability/flammability") are used for flammability and reactivity, and pH is used for scoring corrosivity. Taste/odor and appearance are evaluated within an aesthetics criterion.

- The Sax Toxicity Rating System (Sax and Lewis 1989) includes flammability, reactivity, and explosivity criteria in assigning toxicity ratings to industrial materials.

Among the environmental impacts that have not been included in most current CRS systems are many global and regional issues, such as ozone depleting potential, greenhouse warming, acidification, freshwater eutrophication, photochemical reactivity, etc. Further details pertaining to the use of other endpoints in existing systems are included in the following section.

Incorporating Other Chemical Characteristics in CRS

This section discusses various approaches for incorporating other characteristics in CRS. These characteristics have been divided into 4 categories: chemical properties relating to physical effects or hazards, chemical-environmental interactions, waste reduction and management, and resource productivity.

Chemical properties

Some properties such as vapor pressure (Pv), solubility (S), dissociation constant (pKa), and partition coefficient are discussed in Chapter 2. Other chemical properties described below could be considered for CRS.

Ignitability/flammability

Ignitability refers to the ability of substances to start to burn. Flammability refers to the ability of substances to easily ignite and burn with great rapidity. Several existing ranking systems have included these properties (e.g., Sampaolo and Binetti 1986, 1989; Gjøs et al 1989; Sax and Lewis 1989; ATSDR 1992). In addition, guidance has been provided in U.S. Resource Conservation and Recovery Act (RCRA) by the National Academy of Science (NAS) (*Federal Register* 48, 102 1983) and by the European Union (EU) (67/548/EEC). Scoring systems that have used ignitability and flammability, as well as criteria developed to define ignitability and flammability, were reviewed for this chapter and are described below.

Scoring approaches. Scores for flammability were assigned by the MCMR (MDNR 1987). Very flammable gases and very volatile flammable liquids and chemicals were assigned a score of "1"; other chemicals received a score of "0" if there was insufficient information or "*" if there was no information.

The NFPA (1986) has assigned flammability hazard ratings to many substances according to the following rating system:

Hazard rating	Chemical flammability characteristics
0	will not burn
1	will ignite if preheated
2	will ignite if moderately heated
3	will ignite at most ambient temperatures
4	burns readily at ambient conditions

Sampaolo and Binetti (1986, 1989) assigned scores for flammability on a scale of 0 to 3, based on EEC Directive 67/548, as follows:

Score	Flammability characteristic, based on available data
0	Not flammable gas, liquid or solid
1	Flammable liquid
2	Flammable solid or highly flammable liquid
3	Extremely flammable gas or liquid, or auto-flammable substance

(If data are not available, an assumption is made based on chemical structure and physical state.)

Defining criteria. The MCMR defines very flammable gases and very volatile flammable liquids and chemicals as those that can be ignited under normal temperature conditions. The RCRA considers substances with FPs < 60°C (140°F) to be ignitable substances (e.g., oxidizers and liquids).

A criterion for ignitability was established under Section 102 of the Comprehensive Environmental Response, Compliance & Liability Act – Reportable Quantity (CERCLA-RQ) ranking process. Under the CERCLA-RQ ranking process, the following NAS scale for ignitability was proposed based on FPs (closed cup) and BPs (EMS 1985; USEPA 1989c):

Category	Flash point	Boiling point
Extremely hazardous	<100 °F (37.8 °C)	<100 °F (37.8 °C)
Highly hazardous	<100 °F (37.8 °C)	>100 °F (37.8 °C)
Hazardous	>100–140 °F (37.8–60 °C)	
Slightly hazardous	>140 °F (60 °C)	
Insignificant hazard	Non-combustible	

After the proposal, the U.S. Environmental Protection Agency (USEPA) added a new category, "pyrophoric," for spontaneous ignition and deleted the slightly hazardous and insignificant hazard categories.

The EU proposed the following criteria in a 3-tier system (67/548/EEC):

- Flammable substances (risk phrase 10) are
  - liquids with an FP $\geq 21°C$ and $\leq 55°C$.

- Highly flammable substances (danger symbol "F," risk phrase 11) are
  - substances that may catch fire in contact with air at ambient temperature without application of energy or after brief contact with ignition source,
  - liquids with an FP $< 21°C$,
  - gaseous substances flammable in air at normal pressure, or
  - substances that, in contact with water or steam, evolve highly flammable gases in dangerous quantities.

- Extremely flammable substances (danger symbol "F_x", risk phrase R12) are
  - liquids that have an FP$< 0°C$ and a BP $\leq 35°C$.

Comparison of defining criteria. The criterion, ignition at normal temperature, proposed in the MCMR is comparable to the NAS scale for ignitability (FP $<100°F$ ($37.8°C$), the RCRA criterion of FPs $< 60°C$ ($140°F$), and the EU's criterion of FP $\geq 21°C$ and $\leq 55°C$. This comparability implies that MCMR's very flammable gases and very volatile flammable liquids and chemicals are probably equivalent to the NAS's extremely hazardous substances, RCRA's ignitable substances, and EU's flammable substances. Based on the MCMR system, all these substances would be assigned a score of 1.

Future considerations. The criterion proposed by the EU as well as those proposed under CERCLA and RCRA may be considered in CRS. The following references consider flammability for chemical ranking: Sampaolo and Binetti 1986, 1989; Gjøs et al. 1989; Sax and Lewis 1989; ATSDR 1992. Based on these works, it may be possible to develop criteria and scores for flammable and ignitable substances.

Explosivity

Explosivity refers to the ability of a stable substance to undergo a rapid, exothermic chemical change in the absence of an external source of oxygen.

Scoring approaches. Sampaolo and Binetti (1986, 1989) assigned scores for explosive properties on a scale of 0 to 2, as follows: 0 - not explosive (shock, friction, flame); 2 - explosive (shock, friction, flame). In their scoring approach, if data are not available, an assumption is made based on chemical structure and physical state.

Defining criteria. In EU legislation on "dangerous substances," explosive substances are substances that may explode under the presence of a flame or that are more sensitive to shocks or friction than dinitrobenzene. The EU described dangerous substances using 2 risk phrases:

- "Risk" of explosion by shock, friction, fire, or other sources of ignition (R2). This includes many organic peroxides.
- "Extreme risk" of explosion by shock, friction, fire, or other sources of ignition (R3). This group includes picrates, pentaerythritol tetranitrate (PETN) and dibenzoyl peroxide.

Future considerations. The criteria proposed by the EU may be considered for scoring. The following references consider explosivity for chemical ranking: Sampaolo and Binetti 1986, 1989; Gjøs et al. 1989; Sax and Lewis 1989. After this information is reviewed, it may be possible to develop criteria and scores for explosive substances.

Oxidizing properties

An oxidizing substance, or "oxidant," supports the combustion of another substance, releases oxygen, or removes hydrogen from another substance. In EU legislation, substances with oxidizing properties produce highly exothermic reactions in contact with other substances, particularly flammable substances.

Oxidation was included in a system developed for USEPA's Office of Water to rank Priority Pollutants under Section 307(a) of the Clean Water Act (Cornaby et al. 1986). Sampaolo and Binetti (1986, 1989) assigned scores for oxidizing properties on a scale of 0 to 2, as follows: 0 - not oxidizing; 1 - faintly oxidizing; 2 - oxidizing. In their scoring approach, if data are not available, an assumption is made based on chemical structure and physical state.

Reactivity (instability)

Reactive chemicals are defined in the RCRA as those that are unstable and undergo violent changes without detonating, e.g., chemicals that generate toxic gases on contact with water.

Scoring approaches. The MCMR assigned scores for reactivity. A score of "1" was assigned to chemicals that were "highly reactive." A score of "0" was assigned if there was insufficient information and "*" if there was no information (MDNR 1987). The NFPA assigned reactivity hazard ratings according to the following rating system (NFPA 1986): stable and not reactive with water = 0; unstable if heated = 1; violent chemical change = 2; shock and heat may detonate = 3; may detonate = 3.

Defining criteria. The MCMR defined "highly reactive" chemicals as those that
- violently react with water,
- readily detonate,

- explosively decompose, or
- explosively react at ambient temperature and pressure.

USEPA proposed the following 5-level NAS scale for categories of chemicals that react with water and initiate a self-reaction (*Federal Register* 48, 102 1983):

Category	Water reaction	Self-reaction
Extremely hazardous	e.g., SO_2	explosion or detonation
Highly hazardous	e.g., oleum	polymerization, stabilizer needed
Hazardous	e.g., NH_3, HCl	polymerization if contaminated
Slightly hazardous	e.g., Cl_2	polymerization, low heat
Insignificant hazard	no appreciable reaction	

After proposing the NAS scale, USEPA added a new category, "inflames with water" (e.g., Na, CaC_2) and listed it as the first category before "extremely hazardous."

Future considerations. The criteria proposed by the USEPA may be considered for scoring. The following references consider reactivity for chemical ranking criteria: EMS 1985; Sax and Lewis 1989; USEPA 1989c; ATSDR 1992. After this information is reviewed, it may be possible to develop criteria and scores for reactive substances.

Corrosivity

Corrosivity refers to the ability of a substance to cause metals to degrade (e.g., oxidation of iron to rust) or to destroy body tissues (e.g., destruction of skin by strong acids or bases).

Scoring approaches. Michigan Critical Material Register assigned 3 scores for corrosivity (MDNR 1987). Chemicals with pH ≤ 2 or ≥ 12 received a score of "1", chemicals with pH >2 and <12 received a score of "0" and chemicals with insufficient information an "*".

Defining criteria. Under RCRA a corrosive chemical is
- aqueous with pH <2 or ≥ 12.5, or
- a liquid that corrodes steel at a rate greater than 6.35 mm/year at 55°C (130°F).

Integrating physical effects

Sampaolo and Binetti (1986, 1989) expressed flammability, explosivity, and oxidizing properties as a total risk index (RI) for physical effects:

$$\text{RI, physical effects} = \frac{\text{PCP (flammability + explosivity + oxidizing)} \times \text{QRP}}{\text{maximum possible score}} \times 100\%$$

where

PCP	=	physical–chemical properties;
Q	=	score for quantity on market;
RP	=	score for size of risk population;
flammability	=	score for flammability, on a scale of 0 to 3 (see "Ignitability/flammability");
explosivity	=	score for explosivity, on a scale of 0 to 2 (see "Explosivity"); and
oxidizing	=	score for oxidizing property, on a scale of 0 to 2 (see "Oxidizing properties").

Chemical-environmental interactions

This section describes potential, direct chemical–environmental interactions. Scoring criteria for these direct interactions may be considered for use in some types of CRS systems, where appropriate, because they are widely accepted in the scientific community as causing secondary impacts of concern and because simple scoring procedures exist for evaluating the relative contribution of a specific chemical to one of these impacts. The potential primary impacts discussed in this section are limited to changes to environmental media resulting from chemical releases and are used as surrogates for the secondary impacts (e.g., human health, environmental toxicity, or corrosion of valuable structures) that are more difficult to quantify on an individual chemical basis.

It is important to note that these chemical characteristics reflect, for the most part, new and still developing fields of global-scale environmental science. Their use in CRS could reveal some interesting trends and relationships, provided that this suits the purpose of a particular CRS. It should be recognized that data needed to consider these characteristics in a CRS are quite scarce for most substances. As the state of the science develops, enough data will presumably be generated to permit at least some of these characteristics to be evaluated appropriately and more frequently.

The Interagency Testing Committee (ITC) has scored chemicals for chemical–environmental interactions (Walker 1995). These scores and the rationales for the scores are listed below:

Suspicion of chemical-environmental interactions	Score
Strong	3
Some	2
Few	1
None	0

Greenhouse effect/global warming potential

The earth's temperature is determined by the balance of incoming solar radiation and outgoing infrared radiation (Weubbles and Edmonds 1991; Heijungs et al. 1992a; Nordic Council of Ministers 1992). Chemicals (particularly atmospheric gases) that absorb infrared radiation could lead to an increase in the planet's temperature, an effect known as "global warming" or the "greenhouse effect" (Fava et al. 1993). Global warming potentials (GWP) expressed relative to carbon dioxide (i.e., by defining the GWP for CO_2 as "1") have been developed for important greenhouse gases by the International Panel on Climate Change (IPCC). The GWPs for CH_4 and NO_2 are 11 and 270, respectively, over a 100-year time horizon. Global warming potentials can be estimated for chemicals that do not have published values, by using data in the Atmospheric Oxidation Rate Program available through Syracuse Research Corporation (SRC), Syracuse, New York. This program estimates the gas-phase reaction rate between organic chemicals and hydroxyl radicals, ozone, and nitrate radicals, based on chemical structure.

Scoring example: The following scores for GWPs are based on those by Tolle et al. (1994).

Score	GWP: Equal mass relative to CO_2 over 100 years
1	< 1
3	1–99
5	100–499
7	500–4999
9	> 5000

In Tolle's scheme, a higher score represents a lesser environmental impact. For this chapter, Tolle's scores have been reassigned to be consistent with the majority of schemes in which higher scores represent greater impacts.

Ozone depletion potential

Some chemicals have the potential to deplete ozone from the stratosphere (Heijungs et al. 1992a; Nordic Council of Ministers 1992; Fava et al. 1993), e.g., by reacting with it to produce oxygen. Reduction in the stratospheric ozone layer will cause more biologically harmful ultraviolet (UV-B) radiation to reach the earth's surface. UV-B radiation can increase the incidence of skin cancer and ocular disorders (e.g., cataracts), cause premature skin aging in humans, and increase the incidence of plant diseases (OTA 1991). Impacts of UV-B radiation on plants have been reviewed by Manning and Tiedemann (1995). Ozone depletion potential (ODP) is usually expressed relative to the ozone destruction activity of the chlorofluorocarbons CFC-11 or CFC-12. Ozone depletion potentials can be estimated by using data in the Atmospheric Oxidation Rate Program available through SRC.

Scoring example. The following scores for ODP values are based on those suggested by Tolle et al. (1994):

Score	ODP (relative to CFC-11 & CFC-12)
1	< 0.01
3	0.01–0.39
5	0.40–0.69
7	0.40–0.99
9	≥ 1.00

Photochemical oxidant creation potential

Photochemical oxidants are created as a result of reactions between NO_x and volatile organic compounds (VOCs) or hydrocarbons (HCs) under the influence of UV radiation (Heijungs et al. 1992a; Nordic Council of Ministers 1992). Photochemical oxidants (e.g., ozone) cause atmospheric smog, which causes visibility problems, eye irritation, respiratory tract problems, and crop damage (Fava et al. 1993). Photochemical oxidant creation potential (POCP) is the ratio between the change in ozone concentration 1) due to a change in emission of VOCs or HCs and 2) due to a change in emission of ethylene. The POCP for emissions of different VOCs and HCs have been calculated (Heijungs et al. 1992b).

Scoring example. The following scores for POCPs are based on those suggested by Tolle et al. (1994):

Score	POCP
1	≤ 0.005
3	0.050–0.006
5	0.500–0.051
7	0.999–0.501
9	≥ 1.000

Odor threshold values

An odor threshold value (OTV) is the lowest chemical concentration that can be detected by humans. Odor threshold values do not indicate the quality of the odor, e.g., whether the odor is noxious or fragrant. Scores for OTV may be applicable to chemical production sites, wastewater treatment plants, drinking water, and emissions from materials used in home and commercial construction.

Scoring example. In the MCMR system, a score of "1" is assigned to a chemical that imparts a taste or an odor to fish or to water at concentrations ≤ 0.01 mg/L in at least 2 reports. A score of "0" is assigned if this criterion is not satisfied and a "*" if there are insufficient data.

The MCMR odor/taste scoring system is limited to water. It would be useful to develop a scoring system, based on the OTV, for odor in air. Thus, the following ranking system for OTV is proposed, where a score of "9" indicates the greatest impact:

Score	OTV (mg/m^3)
1	> 10
3	1–10
5	0.1–1
7	0.001–0.1
9	< 0.001

Eutrophication potential

Eutrophication is an increase in algal or plant biomass resulting from addition of mineral nutrients (usually nitrogen or phosphate) to soil or water. Eutrophication potentials (EPs) have been calculated by Heijungs et al. (1992b) based on the average composition of biomass $(C_{106}H_{263}O_{110}N_{16}P)$ relative to phosphate (PO_4^{3-}) for evaluation of the impacts of nutrient release on the environment.

Scoring example. The following is an example of how a CRS could be used to evaluate the EP of an aquatic environment; a score of "9" indicates the greatest environmental impact. Score modifiers are suggested for use if the nutrient sensitivity of the receiving aquatic environment is known or wastewater is treated to remove nutrients:

Score	EP relative to phosphate
9	>3 (P)
7	1–3 (PO_4)
5	0.30–0.99 (N, NH_4)
3	0.10–0.29 (NO, NO_2, NO_x)
1	<0.10
*	Insufficient information

Score Modifiers:

(A) Decrease the score by 4 points (minimum score of 1) if all surface-water bodies likely to receive nutrients via wastewater from the process or life-cycle stage under consideration are known to be relatively insensitive to nutrient additions. Potentially sensitive surface-water bodies are considered to be those with phosphate concentrations greater than 50 g/L for streams at the point where they enter lakes or reservoirs, 25 g/L within lakes or reservoirs, and 100 g/L for streams not discharging to lakes or impoundments (USEPA 1976).

(B) Decrease the score by 2 or 4 points (minimum score of 1) if all wastewater effluents from the process or life-cycle stage under consideration are known to undergo, respectively, secondary or tertiary wastewater treatment before release into water bodies insensitive to nutrient addition. For this modifier, the secondary or tertiary treatment should only be given a debit of 0 or 2 points, respectively, if the treated effluent flows into a sensitive water body (as defined in modifier A).

Acidification potential

The potential of a chemical to contribute to acid precipitation has been documented as a concern by numerous sources (e.g., Heijungs et al. 1992a; Nordic Council of Ministers 1992; Fava et al. 1993). Acid deposition is primarily created by the emission of sulfur and nitrogen compounds (Nordic Council of Ministers 1992). Acid deposition includes both wet deposition (acid rain) by chemical scavenging and deposit via precipitation (rain, snow, fog) and dry deposition by absorption of gases or by particle collection at surfaces (Longcore et al. 1993). Acid deposition is a large-scale regional phenomenon that can involve long-distance transport of sulfur- and nitrogen-containing air pollutants. Potential secondary ecological consequences of acid deposition include changes in surface water chemistry, decline in fish populations, leaching of toxic metals from soils into surface waters, decreased forest growth, increased incidence of plant diseases, and accelerated damage to materials. Much of the bedrock in the northeastern U.S. and Canada contains total alkalinity of less than 200 µg/L and thus lacks acid-neutralizing capacity, making the soil particularly sensitive to acidic deposition. The Adirondack region of New York has the most acidic lakes of any area in the U.S. (Mitchell et al. 1994). One specific concern in this area is the presence of mercury in fish at levels of concern to humans and fish-eating wildlife. The increased availability of mercury, including highly toxic methylmercury, to fish may be the result of acid deposition.

Acidification potential (AP) values have been calculated for chemical air emissions contributing to acid rain, based on the potential amount of H^+ per mass unit relative to the same parameter for SO_2, shown below (Heijungs et al. 1992a).

Species	AP
SO_2	1.00
NO	1.07
NO_2	0.70
NO_x	0.70
NH_3 (NH_4^+)	1.88

Scoring example. Acidification potentials have also been determined for hydrochloric acid and hydrofluoric acid. The following is an example of how AP values could be considered in a CRS, where a score of "9" indicates the greatest environmental impact:

Score	Criteria ranges for AP relative to sulfate
9	≥ 1.50 (HF, NH_3)
7	1.00–1.49 (SO_2, NO)
5	0.50–0.99 (NO_2, NO_x, HCl)
3	0.10–0.49
1	< 0.09
*	Insufficient information

Score modifier:

Decrease the score by 4 points (minimum of 1), if all areas likely to receive acid deposition due to air emissions from the process or life-cycle stage under consideration (i.e., areas downwind of emissions) are known to be relatively insensitive to acid deposition. Areas sensitive to acid deposition are those where the underlying bedrock has a total alkalinity of less than 200 µeq/L. Most of the eastern U.S. and eastern Canada qualify as sensitive to acid deposition using this threshold, as demonstrated by the presence of lakes with a pH of ≤ 5.0 (Longcore et al. 1993). Most of the general effects of acid deposition have been observed to date in the northeastern U.S. (especially the Adirondack region of northern New York) and eastern Canada (e.g., Sudbury, Ontario).

Waste reduction and management

In terms of reducing and effectively managing chemical wastes and releases, arguably the most important criterion in current decision-making by industry is technical and economic feasibility. Therefore, for some CRS applications, it may be appropriate to include measures of feasibility where possible, e.g., a substance's relative treatability.

Scoring example. A potential scoring system for waste treatability has been recommended by Cornaby et al. (1990):

Score	Removal %
5	≤ 60
4	>60–80
3	>80–95
2	>95–99
1	>99

Treatability (destruction and removal efficiency) has been estimated for a variety of chemicals and wastes. For example, data on the treatability of numerous chemical substances in sewage under various treatment plant conditions and technologies have been compiled in the USEPA's Risk Reduction Engineering Laboratory (RREL) Treatability Database (USEPA 1994c). A significant amount of work has also been done to assess feasibility of source reduction and recycling alternatives by USEPA, state technical assistance centers, and others, although it is unknown if this information has been compiled, by chemical or waste stream, in one database.

To develop indices to predict the technical and economic feasibility of source reduction and recycling alternatives for a chemical waste or release, information would be needed not only on the properties of the chemical itself but also on the form of the waste (if the chemical is in a waste matrix such as organic sludge) and on the industry sector and process generating the waste or release. To predict the treatability of chemicals, information on the source would be less important, but additional information on the waste matrix (e.g., pH, solids content, total organic content) would likely be needed. Based on this information, the commercial availability of demonstrated source reduction, recycling, and/or treatment technologies for the chemical/waste/industrial source could be determined and a general yes/no index of feasibility could be developed. This could also be a useful tool for indicating where opportunities lie for developing new or improved treatment technologies. The USEPA is currently exploring the development of this type of general index for RCRA hazardous wastes.

In the European eco-labeling scheme, scoring systems for emission of waste in the life cycle of paper products and the reuse of waste as raw material in new products for building insulation have been introduced.

Resource productivity

Environmental impacts associated with the consumption of natural resources have been recognized in general terms for many years. In the Brundtland Commission's 1987 report, "Our Common Future," the importance of resource productivity for alleviating environmental as well as developmental problems was put into focus on the international political level for the first time. Recently, Schmidt-Bleek (1994) developed a concept for estimating the environmental impact potential of industrial products based on their resource intensity on a life-cycle basis. In this concept, the aggregated inputs of materials and energy for the following are presumed to represent an initial estimate for the environmental impact intensity of products:

- providing materials and energy,
- manufacturing,
- using/applying,
- recycling,
- disposing,
- transporting, and
- packaging products and intermediates.

Because mass and energy are defined by internationally agreed units, ranking of industrial goods — as well as its international harmonization — are built-in features of this concept.

Removing matter from natural deposits or locations affects the ecological equilibria at those locations. Thus, each time coal, steel, gravel, and sand are consumed and each time soil, water, and overburden are moved or redirected by technical means, ecological changes result. Today, humankind moves, converts, and consumes megatons of materials at more than twice the geological rate. The international Factor 10 Club recommended in 1994 that industrialized economies should increase their average resource productivity tenfold or more in order to move decisively toward sustainability. "The technical potential for such a goal over 50 years is enormous" (Factor 10 Club 1994).

At this time, neither sufficient data nor experience are available to allow widespread routine application of the resource productivity concept for ranking industrial goods, including chemicals. Within a few years, this situation may improve. The resource productivity approach will not replace the traditional ecotoxicity approach for assessing and ranking chemicals but will complement it.

Information needed to rank and score chemicals with respect to their relative resource productivity may be generated by obtaining the following information, if possible, in increasing order of complexity:

Step	Increasing level of analysis
0	Production-related material and energy intensity (MI for production)
1	Material and energy for recycling, use, and disposal
2	Material and energy intensity from production to finished product (e.g., to the "manufacturer's gate")
3	Full resource intensity analysis for the whole life cycle
4	Land use intensity for the whole life cycle, mainly in the areas of resource extraction, transportation, and disposal

The following 3 factors related to assessing relative resource productivity are quantifiable, and thus could be incorporated into a CRS, depending on its purpose:

1) energy use,
2) land use, and
3) material resource use.

A significant amount of thought has gone into the latter factor over the last few years, particularly by Schmidt-Bleek (1993).

When material intensities of products are considered, all material inputs must also be considered, including those that occur during mining, manufacturing, use, recycling, and disposing activities as well as in transporting, packaging, and at infrastructural facilities. Not only must material resources that are physically embodied in products be summed but also ancillary material movements such as overburden, use of water, etc. This process is essentially similar to monetary cost accounting.

Lowering the material inputs into the economy results in a commensurate decrease and composition of waste flows, and it also affects the quantity of toxic substances favorably. The dematerialization will also require intensive innovation so as to make more ecological "service delivery machines" (products) available that will not compromise end-use satisfaction. The measure proposed for capturing the specific resource consumption is the material intensity per unit service (MIPS) (Schmidt-Bleek 1993).

Structure and Integration of Other Characteristics into CRS

As discussed in Chapter 1, CRS is often performed in tiers with increasingly sophisticated levels of analysis and increased data as one moves from lower to higher tiers. The tiered approach is often used to screen chemicals to reduce the number of chemicals for which the increasingly sophisticated analysis and increased data needs are necessary. Proposed tiers for the other chemical characteristics discussed in this chapter follow, in an order reflecting decreasing data availability at present:

Tier	Other chemical characteristics
0	Chemical properties
1	Ozone depletion potential Global warming potential Odor threshold analysis
2	Acidification potential Photochemical reactivity Photochemical oxidation creation potential Eutrophication potential
3	Feasibility of treatment of waste Feasibility of source reduction and recycling of waste Resource productivity

To what extent the inclusion of other chemical characteristics (as defined in this chapter) into CRS will influence or be useful in the prioritization of chemicals is not fully known. A trial exercise is needed to determine if scoring/ranking for these characteristics is a vital component of an overall scoring system or is only an adjunct to be used to "fine-tune" the scoring/ranking of chemicals. Many of these "other characteristics" criteria need further development before such an exercise can be conducted. Therefore, once these characteristics have been adequately defined, a subset of chemicals should be identified and evaluated according to each of the characteristics. Chemicals that have previously been scored for health, ecological, and exposure indices would be the best candidates because the added "weight" of "other characteristics" scoring could then be determined.

Summary and Recommendations for Future Work

In summary, important other chemical characteristics include the following:
- chemical properties (e.g., flammability, corrosivity);
- chemical-environmental interaction (e.g., ozone depletion, odor, global warming);
- waste reduction and management (e.g., source reduction, ability to detect chemicals in waste); and
- material resources, energy use, and land use associated with chemical production.

The extent to which these characteristics are incorporated into a CRS system depends on the specific purpose of the particular CRS. Methods for quantifying these characteristics require further development if they are to be used in CRS systems. Some areas are more developed and already used in CRS systems (e.g., physical effects and global/regional impacts), while other areas require further work or research (e.g., waste management and resource productivity).

Recommendations for future work include the following:

- Further develop criteria for evaluating physical–chemical and aesthetic properties (e.g., flammability/ignitability, explosivity/reactivity, oxidation, corrosivity, odor, taste, and clarity).
- Further develop methods to quantify and include alteration-of-environment effects (global warming, ozone depletion, photochemical oxidation, eutrophication, and acidification).
- Improve/develop methods for ranking resource productivity.
- Evaluate the impact of including these other chemical characteristics in a CRS system.

References

Bouwes NW, Hassur SM. 1997. Toxics Release Inventory relative risk-based environmental indicators methodology. Washington DC: U.S. Environmental Protection Agency (USEPA) Office of Pollution, Prevention and Toxics. June.

[AQUIRE] Aquatic Information Retrieval Database. (no date). Duluth MN: U.S. Environmental Protection Agency (USEPA), Office of Research and Development, National Health and Environmental Effects Laboratory, Mid-Continent Ecology Division.

Atkinson R. 1987. A structure-activity relationship for the estimation of rate constants for the gas-phase reactions of OH radicals with organic compounds. *Int J Chem Kinet* 19:799–828.

Atkinson R. 1994. Gas-phase tropospheric chemistry of organic compounds. *J Physical and Chemical Reference Data*. Monograph No. 2. Riverside CA: Statewide Air Pollution Research Center and Department of Soil and Environmental Sciences, University of California.

[ATSDR] Agency for Toxic Substances and Disease Registry. 1992. Support document: the CERCLA 104 priority list of hazardous substances that will be the subject of toxicological profiles. Washington DC: U.S. Public Health Service, Department of Health and Human Services.

Auer CM. 1992. The OECD "SIDS" Program. 17 June 1992 [memorandum updated from OECD document S6/CK/BIAC91.181/4.9.91]. Director, Existing Chemicals Assessment Division. Washington DC: U.S. Environmental Protection Agency (USEPA), Office of Pesticides and Toxic Substances.

Behret H, editor. 1989a. Existing chemicals of environmental relevance. GDCh-Advisory Committee on Existing Chemicals of Environmental Relevance. New York: VCH.

Behret H, editor. 1989b. Existing chemicals of environmental relevance II, selection criteria and second priority list. GDCh-Advisory Committee on Existing Chemicals of Environmental Relevance. New York: VCH .

Bintein S, Devillers J, Karcher W. 1993. Non-linear dependence of fish bioconcentration on n-octanol/ water partition coefficient. *SAR and QSAR in Environmental Research* 1:29–39.

Biobyte Inc. 1996. [computer software: 3 versions currently available as of June 1996]. (1) CLOGP for Windows, Version 1.0; (2) MACLOGP (for Macintosh computers), Version 2.0,; (3) CLOGP P VAX/ VMS, Version 2.10. Claremont CA: Biobyte Inc. Based on research of C. Hansch and A. Leo.

Boethling RS, Howard PH, Meylan W, Stiteler W, Beauman J, Tirado N. 1994. Group contribution method for predicting probability and rate of aerobic biodegradation. *Environ Sci Technol* 28:459–465.

Bouchard D. 1991. Review of Region VII TRI strategy [memorandum]. Kansas City KS: U.S. Environmental Protection Agency (USEPA) Region VII.

Boublik T, Fried V, Hala E. 1984. The vapor pressure of pure substances: selected values of the temperature dependence of the vapor pressures of some pure substances in the normal and low pressure region. Volume 17. Amsterdam, The Netherlands: Elsevier. 626 p.

Briggs GC. 1981. Theoretical and experimental relationships between soil adsorption, octanol-water partition coefficients, water solubilities, bioconcentration factors, and the parachor. *J Agriculture Food Chemistry* 29:1050–1059.

Brooke LT, Call DJ, Geiger DL, Northcott CE, editors. 1984. Acute toxicities of organic chemicals to fathead minnows (*Pimephales promelas*). Volume 1. Superior WI: Center for Lake Superior Environmental Studies, University of Wisconsin-Superior.

Brundtland Commission. 1987. Our common future, World Commission on Environment and Development. Oxford UK: Oxford Univ Pr.

Budavari S, O'Neil MJ, Smith A, Heckelman PE, Kinneary JF, editors. 1996. The Merck Index. 12th ed. Whitehouse Station NJ: Merck.

Clements R, Nabholz JV, Johnson D, Zeeman M. 1993. The use of quantitative structure activity relationships (QSARs) as screening tools in environmental assessment. In: Gorsuch JW, Dwyer FJ, Ingersoll CG, La Point TW, editors. Environmental toxicology and risk assessment, 2nd volume. Philadelphia PA: American Society for Testing and Materials (ASTM). ASTM STP 1216. p. 555–570.

Cornaby BW, Bennett MS, Clement WH, Gavaskar AR, Pickrel CA, Pomeroy SE, Poston TM, Rench JD, Rieske DE, Rogers CJ. 1986. Results of implementation of a chemical ranking system. Prepared by Battelle. Washington DC: U.S. Environmental Protection Agency (USEPA).

Cornaby BW, Tolle DA, Shuey JA, Mower KJ, Kallander DB, Rench JD. 1990. Implementation of a chemical ranking system [draft final report]. Prepared by Battelle. Washington DC: U.S. Environmental Protection Agency (USEPA), Criteria and Standards Division. USEPA Contract No. 68-03-3534, Work Assignment H2-32, Task 3.

Cowan CE, Mackay D, Feijtel TCJ, Van de Meent D, Di Guardo A, Davies J, Mackay N, editors. 1995. The multimedia fate model: a vital tool for predicting the fate of chemicals. Pensacola FL: SETAC Pr.

Crutcher MR, Parker FL. 1990. A classification system for hazardous chemical wastes. Superfund 90, Hazardous Materials Control Research Institutes, 11th Annual National Conference; 1990 Nov 26–28; Washington DC. p 222–225.

Daubert TE, Danner RP. 1989. Data compilation tables of properties of pure compounds. New York NY: Design Institute for Physical Property Data, American Institute of Chemical Engineers.

Davis GA, Swanson M. Jones A. 1994. Comparative evaluation of chemical ranking and scoring methodologies. Knoxville TN: Univ of Tennessee, Center for Clean Products and Clean Technologies.

[EC] European Commission. 1994. Available valid data assessment factors to be applied to the lowest LC50, EC50, or long term NOEC. In: Risk assessment of existing substances, Technical Guidance Document. XI 1919/94-EN.

Ellington JJ, Stancil FE, Payne WD. 1987. Measurement of hydrolysis rate constants for evaluation of hazardous waste land disposal. Volume 1, Data on 32 chemicals. Athens GA: U.S. Environmental Protection Agency (USEPA). Report No. EPA/60/53-86/043.

Emans HJB. 1993. Priority setting of existing chemical substances by means of the IPS-Model. Interim Report II. The Netherlands: National Institute of Public Health and Environmental Protection (RIVM).

[EMS] Environmental Monitoring and Services Inc. 1985. Technical background document to support rule making pursuant to CERCLA Section 102, Volumes 1–2. Prepared for U.S. Environmental Protection Agency. Washington DC: Office of Research and Development, Office of Solid Waste and Emergency Response.

Enslein K, Tomb ME, Lander TR. 1984. Structure-activity models of biological oxygen demand. Proc. Workshop Quant. Struct.-Act. Relat. Rochester NY: Health Des., Inc.

Environment Ontario. 1987. The effluent monitoring priority pollutants list. Ontario, Canada: Ontario Ministry of the Environment, Hazardous Contaminants Coordination Branch. ISBN 0-7729-2784-7.

Environment Ontario. 1988. The effluent monitoring priority pollutants list, 1988 update. Ontario, Canada: Ontario Ministry of the Environment, Hazardous Contaminants Coordination Branch. ISBN 0-7729-5450-X.

Environment Canada and Ontario Ministry of Environment and Energy (OMOEE). 1994. The ARET substance selection process and guidelines. Quebec, Canada: Environment Canada, Protection and Conservation, National Office of Pollution Prevention.

[EU] European Union. 1993. Risk assessment of notified new substances. Technical Guidance Document 93/67/EEC.

Factor 10 Club. 1994. Carnoules Declaration. Wuppertal, Germany: Wuppertal Institute for Climate, Environment and Energy.

Fava J, Consoli F, Denison R, Dickson K, Mohin T, Vigon B, editors. 1993. A conceptual framework for life-cycle impact assessment. Pensacola FL: Society of Environmental Toxicology and Chemistry (SETAC) and SETAC Foundation for Environmental Education, Inc.

Finkel AM. 1990. Confronting uncertainty in risk management, a guide for decision-makers. Washington DC: Center for Risk Management, Resources for the Future.

Foran JA, Glenn BS. 1993. Criteria to identify chemical candidates for sunsetting in the Great Lakes Basin. Washington DC: George Washington Univ, Environmental Health and Policy Program, Dept of Health Care Sciences.

Geiger, DL, Brooke LT, Call DJ, editors. 1990. Acute toxicities of organic chemicals to fathead minnows (*Pimephales promelas*). Volume V. Superior WI: Univ of Wisconsin-Superior, Center for Lake Superior Environmental Studies.

Geiger DL, Call DJ, Brooke LT, editors. 1988. Acute toxicities of organic chemicals to fathead minnows (*Pimephales promelas*). Volume IV. Superior WI: Univ of Wisconsin-Superior, Center for Lake Superior Environmental Studies.

Geiger DL, Northcott CE, Call DJ, Brooke LT, editors. 1985. Acute toxicities of organic chemicals to fathead minnows (*Pimephales promelas*). Volume II. Superior WI: Univ of Wisconsin-Superior, Center for Lake Superior Environmental Studies.

Geiger DL, Poirier SJ, Brooke LT, Call DJ, editors. 1986. Acute toxicities of organic chemicals to fathead minnows (*Pimephales promelas*). Volume III. Superior WI: Univ of Wisconsin-Superior, Center for Lake Superior Environmental Studies.

Gillett JW. 1983. A comprehensive pre-biologic screen for ecotoxicologic effects. *Environ Toxicol Chem* 2:463–476.

Gjøs N, Møller M, Hœgh GS, Kolset K. 1989. Existing chemicals: systematic data collection and handling for priority setting. Oslo, Norway: Center for Industrial Research. Copenhagen, Denmark: Nordic Council of Ministers.

Gustafsson L, Ljung E. 1990. Substances and preparations dangerous for the environment: a system for classification, labelling and safety data sheets. Final Report from a Nordic Working Group. Copenhagen, Denmark: Nordic Council of Ministers.

Haaf, W. 1995. Personal communication with Bill Haaf. DuPont, Wilmington DE.

Haaf, W. 1997. Personal communication with Bill Haaf. DuPont, Wilmington DE.

Hamrick, K.J., H.P. Kollig and A. Bartell. 1992. Computerized extrapolation of hydrolysis rate data. *J Chemical Information and Computer Science* 32:511–514.

Hansch C, Leo AJ. 1987. The Log P data base. Claremont CA: Pomona College.

Hansen BG. 1993. Priority setting using the EPS method: From IUCLID to IPS ranking [draft]. Doc XI/ECB/883/93 (rev.1).

Health Designs Inc. 1990. TOPKAT [computer program]. Rochester NY.

Heidorn, CJA, Hansen BG, Nørager, O. 1996. IUCLID: A database on chemical substances infomation as a tool for the EU-Risk-Assessment-Program. *J Chem Inf Comput Sci* 36:949–954.

Heijungs R, Guinée JB, Huppes G, Lankreijer RM, Udo de Haes HA, Wegener Sleeswijk A, Ansems AMM, Eggels PG, van Duin R, de Goede HP. 1992a. Environmental life cycle assessment of products: backgrounds - October 1992. Leiden, The Netherlands: Center of Environmental Science, Leiden Univ.

Heijungs R, Guinée JB, Huppes G, Lankreijer RM, Udo de Haes HA, Wegener Sleeswijk A, Ansems AMM, Eggels PG, van Duin R, de Goede HP. 1992b. Environmental life cycle assessment of products: guide, October 1992. Leiden, The Netherlands: Center of Environmental Science, Leiden Univ.

Hine J, Mookerjee PK. 1975. The intrinsic hydrophilic character of organic compounds. Correlations in terms of structural contributions. *J Org Chem* 40:292–298.

Hoffman III WF. 1997. Recent advances in Design for Environment at Motorola. *J Industrial Ecology* 1:131–140.

Horvath AL. 1982. Halogenated hydrocarbons: solubility-miscibility with water. New York NY: Marcel Dekker. 889 p.

Howard PH, editor. 1989. Handbook of environmental fate and exposure data for organic chemicals. Volume I, Large production and priority pollutants. Chelsea MI: Lewis.

Howard PH, editor. 1990. Handbook of environmental fate and exposure data for organic chemicals. Volume II, Solvents. Chelsea MI: Lewis.

Howard PH, editor. 1991. Handbook of environmental fate and exposure data for organic chemicals. Volume III, Pesticides. Chelsea MI: Lewis.

Howard PH, editor. 1992. Handbook of environmental fate and exposure data for organic chemicals. Vol. IV, Solvents II. Chelsea MI: Lewis.

Howard PH, Heuber AE, Boethling RS. 1987. Biodegradation data evaluation for structure/biodegradability relations. *Environ Toxicol Chem* 6:1–10.

Howard PH, Hueber AE, Mulesky BC, Crisman JS, Meylan W, Crosbie E, Gray DA, Sage GW, Howard DP, LaMacchia A, Boethling R, Troast R. 1986. BIOLOG, BIODEG and FATE/EXPOS: New files on microbial degradation and toxicity as well as environmental fate/exposure of chemicals. *Environ Toxic Chem* 5:977–988.

[HSDB] Hazardous Substances Data Bank. Updated periodically. Bethesda MD: MEDLARS Online Information Retrieval System, National Library of Medicine, Toxicology Data Network (TOXNET).

[IARC] International Agency for Research on Cancer. 1987. Updating of IARC Monographs Vol. 1–42, Supplement 7. Lyon, France: World Health Organization.

[IJC] International Joint Commission's Binational Objective Development Committee. 1989. The Great Lakes Water Quality Agreement standard methods and Annex 1, lists of substances. Chicago IL and Toronto, Ontario: IJC.

Jury WA, Spencer WF, Farmer WJ. 1983. Behavior assessment model for trace organics in soil. I. Model description. *J Environ Qual* 12(4):558–564.

Kincaid LE, Bartmess JE. 1993. Evaluation of TRI releases in Indiana, Louisiana, Ohio, Tennessee and Texas. Knoxville TN: Univ of Tennessee, Center for Clean Products and Clean Technologies.

Kincaid LE, Meline JD, Davis GA. 1996. Cleaner technologies substitutes assessment: a methodology and resource guide. Washington DC: U.S. Environmental Protection Agency (USEPA) Office of Pollution Prevention and Toxics. EPA 744-R-95-002.

Klein W, Kördel W, Klein AW, Kuhnen-Clausen D, Weiss M. 1988. Systematic approach for environmental hazard ranking of new chemicals. *Chemosphere* 17:1445–1462.

Klopman G. 1984. Artificial intelligence approach to structure-activity studies. Computer automated structure evaluation of biological activity of organic molecules. *J Am Chem Soc* 106:7313–7321.

Klopman G, Zhang Z, Balthasar DM, Rosenkranz HS. 1995. Computer-automated predictions of aerobic biodegradation of chemicals. *Environ Toxicol Chem* 14:395–403.

Kollig HP. 1993. Environmental fate constants for organic chemicals under consideration for USEPA's Hazardous Waste Identification Projects. Athens GA: U.S. Environmental Protection Agency (USEPA) Environmental Research Laboratory. USEPA/600/R-93/132.

Könemann H, Visser R. 1988. Selection of chemicals with high hazard potential: Part 1: WMS-Scoring System. *Chemosphere* 17:1905–1919.

Larson RJ, Cowan CE. 1995. Quantitative application of biodegradation data to environmental risk and exposure assessments. *Environ Toxicol Chem* 14:1433–1442.

Layton DW, Mallon BJ, Rosenblatt DH, Small MJ. 1987. Deriving allowable daily intakes for systemic toxicants lacking chronic toxicity data. *Reg Toxicol & Pharmacol* 7:96–112.

Lewis DFV, Ioannides C, Parke DV. 1993. Prediction of the carcinogenic potential by computer-optimized molecular parametric analysis of chemical toxicity (COMPACT) via cytochrome P450 interactions. *Poly Arm Cmpds* 3:719–724.

Longcore JR, Boyd H, Brooks RT, Haramis GM, McNicol DK, Newman JR, Smith KA, Stearns F. 1993. Acidic depositions: effects on wildlife and habitats. Bethesda MD: The Wildlife Society. Wildl. Soc. Tech Rev. 93-1. 42 p.

Lyman WJ, Reehl WF. Rosenblatt DH. 1990. Handbook of chemical property estimation methods. Washington DC: American Chemical Society.

Mabey W, Mill T. 1978. Critical review of hydrolysis of organic compounds in water under environmental conditions. *J Phys Chem Ref Data* 7:383–415.

Mackay D, Shiu WY. 1981. A critical review of Henry's Law constants for chemicals of environmental interest. *J Phys Chem Ref Data* 19:1175–99.

Mackay D, Shiu WY, Ma KC. 1992. Illustrated handbook of physical-chemical properties and environmental fate for organic chemicals. Volumes 1–4. Boca Raton FL: Lewis.

Mackay D. 1991. Multimedia environmental models, the fugacity approach. Chelsea MI: Lewis.

Manning WJ, Tiedemann AV. 1995. Climate change: Potential effects of increased atmospheric carbon dioxide (CO_2), ozone (O_3), and ultraviolet-B (UV-B) radiation on plant diseases. *Environ Pollut* 88:219–245.

McNamara BP. 1971. Concepts in health evaluation of commercial and industrial chemicals, long-term versus short-term toxicity tests. In: Mehlman MA, Shapiro RE, Blumenthal H, editors. Advances in modern toxicology. New York NY: Hemisphere, J Wiley. p 61–140.

[MDNR] Michigan Department of Natural Resources. 1987. Critical materials register (criteria and support documents). Lansing MI: MDNR.

Meylan WM, Howard PH, Boethling RS. 1992. Molecular topology/fragment contribution method for predicting soil sorption coefficients. *Environ Sci Technol* 26:1560–1567.

Meylan WM, Howard PH. 1991. Bond contribution method for estimating Henry's Law constants. *Environ Toxicol Chemistry* 10:1283–93.

Meylan WM, Howard PH. 1993. Computer estimation of the atmospheric gas-phase reaction rate of organic compounds with hydroxyl radicals and ozone. *Chemosphere* 20:2293–2299.

Meylan WM, Howard PH. 1995. Atom/Fragment contribution method for estimating octanol-water partition coefficients. *J Pharm Sci* 84:83–92.

Meylan WM, Howard PH, Boethling RS. 1996. Improved method for estimating water solubility from octanol/water partition coefficient. *Environ Toxicol Chem* 15: 100–106.

Mitchell MJ, Driscoll CT, Porter JH, Raynal DJ, Schaefer D, White EH. 1994. The Adirondack Manipulation and Modeling Project (AMMP): design and preliminary results. *Forest Ecology Management* 68(1):87–100. ISSN: 0378-1127.

Nabholz JV, Clements R, Zeeman M, Osborn KC, Wedge R. 1993. Validation of structure activity relations used by the Office of Pollution Prevention and Toxics for the environmental hazard assessment of industrial chemicals. In: JW Gorsuch, FJ Dwyer, Ingersoll CG, La Point TW, editors. Environmental toxicology and risk assessment: 2nd Volume. Philadelphia PA: American Society for Testing and Materials (ASTM). ASTM STP 1216. p 571–590.

National Academy of Sciences. 1983. Risk assessment in the federal government. Washington DC: National Academy Pr.

Neimi GJ, Veith GD, Regal RR, Vaishnav DD. 1987. Structural features associated with degradable and persistent chemicals. *Environ Toxicol Chem* 6:515–527.

[NFPA] National Fire Protection Association. 1986. Recommended system for identification of the fire hazards of materials. Section 704, Fire protection guide on hazardous materials. 9th ed. Quincy MA: NFPA.

[NIOSH] National Institute for Occupational Safety and Health. 1988. National occupational exposure survey. Department of Health and Human Services (NIOSH) Publication No. 88-106. March 1988.

[NIOSH] National Institute for Occupational Safety and Health. 1990. National occupational exposure survey. Department of Health and Human Services (NIOSH) Publication No. 89-102. February 1990.

[NLM] National Library of Medicine. 1986. Toxicology Information On-Line (TOXLINE) [computer database]. Bethesda MD: NLM.

Nordic Council of Ministers. 1992. Product life cycle assessment - principles and methodology. Copenhagen, Denmark: Nordic Council of Ministers. NORD 1992:9.

O'Bryan TR, Ross RH. 1988. Chemical scoring system for hazard and exposure identification. *J Toxicol Env Health* 1:119–34.

[OECD] Organization for Economic Cooperation and Development. 1993–1994. Guidelines for the testing of chemicals. Brussels: OECD.

[OECD] Organization for Economic Cooperation and Development. 1994. USEPA/EC joint project on the evaluation of (quantitative) structure activity relationships (QSARs). Paris: OECD Environment Monographs No. 88.

[OMOE] Ontario Ministry of the Environment. 1990. Ontario MOE Scoring System. Toronto, Ontario: Ontario Ministry of Environment, Hazardous Contaminants Coordination Branch.

[OMOEE] Ontario Ministry of the Environment and Energy. 1994. TOMCAT [computer database]. Version 2.0. Toronto, Canada: OMOEE.

[OTA] Office of Technology Assessment, Congress of the United States. 1991. Changing by degrees: steps to reduce greenhouse gases. Washington DC: U.S. Government Printing Office. OTA-O-482.

Ramsar Convention on Wetlands of International Importance. 1976. International convention for the identification and protection of sensitive wetlands of international importance. (Secretariat based in Gland, Switzerland under the auspices of the United Nations Educational, Scientific and Cultural Organization [UNESCO]; 685 sites worldwide as of 1996; treaty signed by 80 nations.)

Riddick JA, Bunger WB, Sakano TK. 1986. Techniques of chemistry. Volume II, Organic solvents. 4th ed. New York NY: Wiley-Interscience.

Russom CL. 1994. ASTER: ASsessment Tools for the Evaluation of Risk. Version 1.0, a user's guide. Duluth MN: USEPA National Health and Environmental Effects Research Laboratory, Mid-Continent Ecology Division.

Saaty TL. 1980. The analytical hierarchy process. New York NY: McGraw-Hill.

Sampaolo A, Binetti R. 1986. Elaboration of a practical method for priority selections and risk assessment among existing chemicals. *Reg Toxicol Pharmacol* 6:129–154.

Sampaolo A, Binetti R. 1989. Improvement of a practical method for priority selections and risk assessments among existing chemicals. *Reg Toxicol Pharmacol* 10:185–195.

Sangster J. 1993. LOGKOW databank. Montréal PQ, Canada: Sangster Research Laboratories.

Sax NI, Lewis RJ. 1989. Dangerous properties of industrial materials. New York NY: Van Nostrand Reinhold.

Schmidt-Bleek F. 1993. MIPS re-visited. *Fresenius Environ Bull* 2:407–412. (Special issue to p 490).

Schmidt-Bleek F. 1994. Wieviel Umwelt braucht der Mench? MIPS das Mass für Ökologisches Wirtschaften. Germany: Birkhauser Verlag.

Shiu WY, Mackay D. 1986. A critical review of aqueous solubilities, vapor pressure, Henry's law constants, octanol-water partition coefficients of the polychlorinated biphenyls. *J Phys Chem Ref Data 15:911–29.*

Shiu WY, Ma KC, Mackay D, Seiber JN, Wauchope RD. 1990. Solubilities of pesticides chemicals in water. II: Data compilation. *Rev Environ Contam Toxicol* 116:15–187.

Socha, A.C., R. Aucoin, T. Dickie, R. Angelow, and P. Kauss. 1993. *Candidate Substances for Bans, Phase-Outs or Reductions - Multimedia Revision.* Ontario Ministry of Environment and Energy, Toronto, Ontario. ISBN 0-7778-0774-2.

Socha AC, Dickie T, Aucoin R, Angelow R, Kauss P, Rutherford G. 1992. Candidate substances list for bans or phase-outs. Toronto, Ontario: Ontario Ministry of the Environment.

[SRC] Syracuse Research Corporation. 1994. Environmental Fate Data Base (EFDB). PC and on-line versions available. Syracuse NY.

[SRC] Syracuse Research Corporation. 1996. Estimation Programs Interface (EPI©). Version 2.0E. Syracuse NY.

Steen, B. and S.O. Ryding. 1992. *The EPS Enviro-Accounting Method.* Swedish Environmental Research Institute (IVL), Göteborg, Sweden.

Swanson, M.B., Davis, G.A., L. Kincaid, M. B. Swanson, T. Schultz, J. Bartmess, and S. Jones. 1997. Chemical hazard evaluation for management strategies: a method for ranking and scoring chemicals by potential human health and environmental impacts. *Environ Toxicol Chem* In press.

Timmer M, Könemann H, Visser R. 1988. Selection of chemicals with high hazard potential. Part 2: WMS-Scoring System. *Chemosphere* 17:1921–1934.

Tolle DA, Vigon BW, Becker JR, Salem MA. 1994. Development of a pollution prevention factors methodology based on life-cycle assessment: lithographic printing case study. Columbus OH: Battelle. EPA/600/R-94/157.

[USBLS] U.S. Bureau of Labor Statistics. 1995. Employment and wages annual averages, 1995. Washington DC: U.S. Department of Labor, Bureau of Labor Statistics. BLS Bulletin 2483.

U.S. Congress. 1995. Screening and testing chemicals in commerce. Background paper. Washington DC: Office of Technology Assessment. OTA-BP-ENV-166.

[USEPA] U.S. Environmental Protection Agency. 1976. Quality criteria for water. Washington DC: USEPA.

[USEPA] U.S. Environmental Protection Agency. 1978. Measuring air quality: the new pollutants standards index. Washington DC: USEPA Office of Policy Analysis.

[USEPA] U.S. Environmental Protection Agency. 1984a. Framework for risk assessment and risk management. Washington DC: USEPA Office of Policy, Planning, and Evaluation.

[USEPA] U.S. Environmental Protection Agency. 1984b. Estimating "concern levels" for concentrations of chemical substances in the environment. Washington DC: USEPA Office of Toxic Substances, Health and Environmental Review Division, Environmental Effects Branch.

[USEPA] U.S. Environmental Protection Agency. 1986. Superfund public health evaluation manual. Washington DC: Office of Emergency and Remedial Response. EPA/540/1-86/060. October.

[USEPA] U.S. Environmental Protection Agency. 1989b. Risk assessment guidance for Superfund. Volume I, Human health evaluation manual. Washington DC: USEPA Office of Emergency and Remedial Response. EPA/540/1-89/002.

[USEPA] U.S. Environmental Protection Agency. 1989c. Technical background document to support rule making pursuant to CERCLA Section 102. Volume 3. Washington DC: USEPA Office of Solid Waste and Emergency Response.

[USEPA] U.S. Environmental Protection Agency. 1991. National emission standards for hazardous air pollutants for source categories: proposed regulations governing compliance extensions for early reductions of hazardous air pollutants. (Criteria for identifying high risk pollutants). 40 CFR Part 63.

[USEPA] U.S. Environmental Protection Agency. 1992a. Guidelines for exposure assessment. *Federal Register*, Vol. 57, No. 104:22888–22938. Washington DC: USEPA Office of Health and Environmental Assessment.

[USEPA] U.S. Environmental Protection Agency. 1992b. Dermal exposure assessment: principles and applications. Interim report. Washington DC: USEPA Office of Research and Development. EPA-600-8-91-011B. January.

[USEPA] U.S. Environmental Protection Agency. 1992c. Inventory of exposure-related data systems sponsored by federal agencies. Washington DC: USEPA Office of Health Research. EPA/600/R-92/078.

[USEPA] U.S. Environmental Protection Agency. 1992d. MIXTOX: An information system on toxicologic interactions for the MS-DOS personal computer. Version 1.5, User's Guide. Cincinnati OH: USEPA Environmental Criteria and Assessment Office.

[USEPA] U.S. Environmental Protection Agency. 1993a. Chemical use clusters scoring methodology. Washington DC: USEPA Office of Pollution Prevention and Toxics, Chemicals Engineering Branch.

[USEPA] U.S. Environmental Protection Agency. 1993b. Wildlife exposure factors handbook. Washington DC: USEPA Office of Research and Development, Office of Health and Environmental Assessment. EPA/600/R-93/187a,b.

[USEPA] U.S. Environmental Protection Agency. 1994a. Waste minimization national plan. Washington DC: USEPA Office of Solid Waste and Emergency Response. EPA/530-R-94-045.

[USEPA] U.S. Environmental Protection Agency. 1994b. A computer program for estimating the ecotoxicity of industrial chemicals based on structure activity relationships (ECOSAR). Washington DC: USEPA Office of Pollution Prevention and Toxics.

[USEPA] U.S. Environmental Protection Agency. 1994c. Treatability data base. Version 5.0. Cincinnati OH: Risk Reduction Engineering Laboratory.

[USEPA] U.S. Environmental Protection Agency. 1994d. USEPA/EC joint project on the evaluation of quantitative structure activity relationships. Washington DC: USEPA Office of Prevention, Pesticides and Toxic Substances. EPA 743-R-94-001.

[USEPA] U.S. Environmental Protection Agency. 1995a. Compilation of air pollutant emission factors. Volume I. Stationary point and area sources. 5th ed. AP-42. Research Triangle Park NC: USEPA Office of Air Quality Planning and Standards, January 1995.

[USEPA] U.S. Environmental Protection Agency. 1995b. Health effects summary tables, FY1995 annual update. USEPA Office of Solid Waste and Emergency Response. EPA/540/5-95/636.

[USEPA] U.S. Environmental Protection Agency. 1995c. Design for the Environment: building partnerships for environmental improvement. Washington DC: USEPA Office of Pollution Prevention and Toxics. September. EPA/600/K-93/002.

[USEPA] U.S. Environmental Protection Agency. 1996. Proposed guidelines for carcinogen risk assessment. *Federal Register*, Vol. 51, No. 185. September.

[USEPA] U.S. Environmental Protection Agency. 1997a. Waste Minimization Prioritization Tool, Beta test version 1.0, User's guide and system documentation. Draft. Washington DC: USEPA Office of Solid Waste and Emergency Response. June. EPA 530-R-97-019.

[USEPA] U.S. Environmental Protection Agency. 1997b. Integrated risk information system (IRIS) Bethesda MD: National Technical Information Service (NTIS).

van de Meent D. 1993. SimpleBOX: a generic multi-media fate evaluation model. Bilthoven, The Netherlands. RIVM Report No. 6727200001.

van der Zandt PTJ, van Leeuwen CJ. 1992. A proposal for priority setting of existing chemical substances. The Netherlands: Ministry of Housing, Physical Planning and the Environment.

Venman BC, Flaga C. 1985. Development of an acceptable factor to estimate chronic end points from acute toxicity data. *Toxicol Ind Health* 1:261–269.

Verhaar HJ, van Leeuwen CJ, Hermens JL. 1992. Classifying environmental pollutants: structure-activity relationships for predicting aquatic toxicity. *Chemosphere* 25:471–491.

Vermeire TG, van de Zandt PTJ, Roelfzeme H, van Leeuwen CJ. 1994. Uniform system for the evaluation of substances I: principles and structure. *Chemosphere* 29:23–38.

Vieth GD, Defoe DL, Bergstedt BV. 1979. Measuring and estimating the bioconcentration factor of chemicals in fish. *J Fish Res Board Can* 36:1040–1048.

Walker JD, Brink RH. 1989. New cost-effective, computerized approaches to selecting chemicals for priority testing consideration. In: GW Suter II, Lewis MA, editors. Aquatic toxicology and environmental fate: 11th Volume. Philadelphia PA: American Society for Testing and Materials (ASTM). ASTM STP 1007. p 507–536.

Walker JD. 1991. Chemical selection by the TSCA Interagency Testing Committee: use of computerized substructure searching to identify chemical groups for health effects, chemical fate and ecological effects testing. *Sci Total Environ* 109/110:691–700.

Walker JD. 1993a. The TSCA Interagency Testing Committee, 1977 to 1992: Creation, structure, functions and contributions. In: Gorsuch JW, Dwyer FJ, Ingersoll CG, La Point TW, editors. Environmental toxicology and risk assessment: 2nd Volume. Philadelphia PA: American Society for Testing and Materials (ASTM). ASTM STP 1216. p 451–509.

Walker JD. 1993b. The TSCA Interagency Testing Committee's approaches to screening and scoring chemicals and chemical groups: 1977–1983. In: Lu PY, editor. Access and use of information resources in assessing health risks from chemical exposure. Oak Ridge TN: Oak Ridge National Laboratories. p 77–93.

Walker JD. 1995. Estimation methods used by the TSCA Interagency Testing Committee to prioritize chemicals for testing: exposure and biological effects scoring and structure activity relationships. *Toxicology Modeling* 1:123–141.

Walker JD, Whittaker C, McDougal JN. 1996. Role of the TSCA Interagency Testing Committee in meeting the U.S. Government's data needs: designating chemicals for percutaneous absorption testing. In: Marzulli F, Maibach H, editors. Dermatoxicology. Washington DC: Taylor & Francis. p 371–381.

Wauchope RD, Buttler TM, Hornsby AG, Burt Augustijn-Beckers JP. 1992. The SCS/ARS/CES pesticide properties database for environmental decision-making. *Rev Environ Contam Toxicol* 123:1–164.

Weil CS, McCollister DD. 1963. Relationship between short- and long-term feeding studies in designing an effective toxicity test. *Agr Food Chain* 11(6):486–491.

Weil CS, Woodside MD, Benard JR, Carpenter CP. 1969. Relationship between single-peroral, one-week, and ninety-day rat feeding studies. *Toxicol Applied Pharmacol* 14:426–431.

Weininger D, Weininger A, Weininger JL. 1986. SMILES: Simplified Molecular Line Input System - a chemical notation "language" for describing molecular structures in a single-line format, designed for use with computers. *Chem Designs Automation News* 1(8):2–15.

Wuebbles DJ, Edmonds J. 1991. Primer on greenhouse gases. Chelsea MI: Lewis.

Yalkowsky SH, editor. 1989. Arizona database of aqueous solubility. Tucson AZ: Univ of Arizona.

Zeeman M. 1995. Ecotoxicity testing and estimation methods developed under Section 5 of the Toxic Substances Control Act (TSCA). In: Rand G, editor. Fundamentals of aquatic toxicology: effects, environmental fate, and risk assessment. 2nd ed. Washington DC: Taylor and Francis. Chapter 23, p 707–715.

Zeeman M, Auer CM, Clements RG, Nabholz JB, Boethling RS. 1995. USEPA regulatory perspectives on the use of QSAR for new and existing chemical evaluations. *SAR & QSAR in Environ Res* 3(3):179–202.

Zeeman M, Fairbrother A, Gorsuch JW. 1995. Environmental toxicology: testing and screening. Chapter 7, Screening and testing chemicals in commerce. Washington DC: U.S. Congress, Office of Technology Assessment. OTA-BP-ENV-166. p 59–67.

Zeeman M, Gilford J. 1993. Ecological hazard evaluation and risk assessment under EPA's Toxic Substances Control Act (TSCA): an introduction. In: Landis WG, Hughes JS, Lewis MA, editors. Environmental toxicology and risk assessment. Philadelphia PA: American Society for Testing and Materials (ASTM). ASTM STP 1179. p 7-21.

Zeeman M, Nabholz JV, Clements R. 1993. The development of SAR/QSAR for use under USEPA's Toxic Substances Control Act: an introduction. In: Gorsuch JW, Dwyer FJ, Ingersoll CG, La Point TW, editors. Environmental toxicology and risk assessment: 2nd volume. Philadelphia PA: American Society for Testing and Materials (ASTM). ASTM STP 1216. p 523–539.

Bibliography

Examples of additional chemical ranking and scoring methods (not cited in the text):

Abt Associates, Inc., 1991. Ranking the relative hazards of industrial discharges to POTWs and surface waters. Washington DC: U.S. Environmental Protection Agency (USEPA) Office of Policy Analysis.

Beckvar N, Harris L. 1992. Coastal hazardous waste site review, September, 1992. Hazardous materials response and assessment division. Seattle WA: National Oceanic and Atmospheric Administration (NOAA), ORCA.

[DOD] U.S. Department of Defense. 1992. User's manual for the Defense Priority Model (FY 93 version, Interim Draft). Prepared by Earth Technology Corporation and ERM Program Management Company, for U.S. Department of Defense, Office of Deputy Assistant Secretary of Defense (Environment), Washington DC.

Droppo Jr JG, Strenge DL, Buck JW, Hoopes BL, Brockhaus RD, Walter MB, Whelan G. 1989. Multimedia environmental pollutant assessment system application guidance. Volume 2, Guidelines for evaluating MEPAS input parameters. Richland WA: Battelle Memorial Institute, Pacific Northwest Laboratory,.

Halfon E, Reggiani MG. 1986. Notes on ranking chemicals for environmental hazard. *Environ Sci Technol* 20:1173–1179.

Hallstedt PA, Puskar MA, Levine SP. 1986. Application of the hazard ranking system to the prioritization of organic compounds identified at hazardous waste remedial action sites. *Hazardous Waste and Hazardous Materials* 3(2):221–232.

ICF Incorporated. 1990. Targeting pollution prevention opportunities using the 1988 Toxics Release Inventory. Washington DC: U.S. Environmental Protection Agency (USEPA) Office of Policy, Planning and Evaluation, Pollution Prevention.

Jones TD, Walsh PJ, Watson AP, Owen BA, Barnthouse LW, Sanders DA. 1988. Chemical scoring by a rapid screen of hazard (RASH) method. *Risk Analysis* 8(1):99–118.

Laskowski PA, Goring CAI, McCall PJ, Swann RL. 1982. Principles of environmental risk analysis: terrestrial environment. In: Conway R, editor. Environmental risk analysis for chemicals. New York NY: Van Nostrand Reinhold. p 198–240.

Poston TM, Prohammer LA. 1985. A ranking system for Clean Water Act Section 307(a) list of priority pollutants. Prepared by Battelle for U.S. Environmental Protection Agency (USEPA), Washington DC.

Radian Corporation. 1990. The source category ranking system: development and methodology. Research Triangle Park NC: U.S. Environmental Protection Agency (USEPA) Office of Air Quality Planning Standards, Chemicals and Petroleum Branch.

Strenge DC, Peterson SR, Sager S. 1989. Chemical data base for the Multimedia Environmental Pollutant Assessment System (MUSEPAS): Version 1. Richland WA: U.S. Department of Energy, Battelle Memorial Institute, Pacific Northwest Laboratory.

[USEPA] U.S. Environmental Protection Agency. 1986. Screening procedure for chemicals of importance to the Office of Water. Washington DC: U.S. Environmental Protection Agency (USEPA) Office of Health and Environmental Assessment.

[USEPA] U.S. Environmental Protection Agency. 1993. Hazardous air pollutants: proposed regulations governing constructed, reconstructed and modified major sources (40 CFR Part 63).

[USEPA] U.S. Environmental Protection Agency. date unknown. Screening methodology for pollution prevention targeting. U.S. Environmental Protection Agency (USEPA) Office of Toxic Substances.

[USEPA] U.S. Environmental Protection Agency, date unknown. TSCA's TRI chemical risk assessment pre-screening methodology. U.S. Environmental Protection Agency (USEPA) Office of Toxic Substances, Existing Chemical Assessment Division.

Weiss M, Kördel W, Kuhnen-Clausen D, Lange AW, Klein W. 1988. Priority setting of existing chemicals. *Chemosphere* 17:1419–1443.

Whelan G, Buck JW, Strenge DL, Droppo Jr JG, Hoopes BL, Aiken RJ. 1992. Overview of the Multimedia Environmental Pollutant Assessment System (MEPAS). *Hazardous Waste & Hazardous Materials* 9(2):191–208.

Whelan G, Strenge DL, Droppo Jr JG, Steelman BL. 1987. The Remedial Action Priority System (RAPS): mathematical formulations. Richland WA: U.S. Department of Energy, Battelle Memorial Institute, Pacific Northwest Laboratory.

Documents that include a survey or evaluation of chemical ranking and scoring systems:

Abt Associates Inc. 1992. Toxics Release Inventory environmental indicators methodology [draft report]. Washington DC: U.S. Environmental Protection Agency (USEPA) Office of Pollution Prevention and Toxics.

Davis GA, Jones SL. 1993. Critical issues in the development of human health and environmental risk ranking and scoring systems. Presented for the Workshop on Identifying the Framework for the Future of Human Health and Environmental Risk Ranking; 30 June–1 July 1993; Washington DC.

Davis GA, Swanson MB, Jones SL. 1994. Comparative evaluation of chemical ranking and scoring methodologies. Knoxville TN: Univ of Tennessee, Center for Clean Products and Clean Technologies

Environ Corporation. 1986. Examination of the severity of toxic effects and recommendation of a systematic approach to rank adverse effects. Cincinnati OH: U.S. Environmental Protection Agency (USEPA), Office of Environmental Criteria and Assessment.

Foran JA, Glenn BS. 1993. Criteria to identify chemical candidates for sunsetting in the Great Lakes Basin. Washington DC: George Washington Univ, Environmental Health and Policy Program, Department of Health Care Sciences.

Hushon JM, Kornreich MR. 1984. Scoring systems for hazard assessment. In: Saxena J, editor. Volume 3, Hazard assessment of chemicals: current developments. Orlando FL: Academic Pr.

ICF Incorporated. 1993. Summary and comparison of five chemical scoring systems. Submitted to Chemical Manufacturers Association, Washington DC.

ICF Incorporated. 1994. Summary and evaluation of the UT chemical ranking system. Submitted to Chemical Manufacturers Association, Washington DC.

[OECD] Organization for Economic Cooperation and Development . 1986. Existing chemicals: systematic investigation, priority setting and chemicals reviews. Paris, France.

Waters RD, Crutcher MR, Parker FL. 1993. Hazard ranking systems for chemical wastes and chemical waste sites. In: Saxena J, editor. Volume 8, Hazard assessment of chemicals. Washington DC: Taylor and Francis.

Other Related Documents

Ashby J, Doerrer NG, Flamm FG, Harris JE, Hughes DH, Johannsen FR, Lewis SC, Krivanek ND, McCarthy JF, Moolenaar RJ, Raabe GK, Reynolds RC, Smith JM, Stevens JT, Teta MJ, Wilson JD. 1990. A scheme for classifying carcinogens. *Regulatory Toxicol Pharmacol* 12:270–295.

Bayer E, Fleischhauer G. 1994. II Status report on the testing activities according to the German program for existing chemicals. *Chemosphere* 29(2):201–239.

[CLC] Canadian Labor Congress. 1992. A critique of the Ontario hazard assessment system. Ottawa Canada: CLC Environment Bureau.

Clements RG, Nabholtz JV, Johnson DW, Zeeman M. 1993. The use and application of QSARs in the Office of Toxic Substances for ecological hazard assessment of new chemicals. In: Environmental toxicology and risk assessment. Philadelphia PA: American Society for Testing and Materials (ASTM). ASTM STP 1179.

Freij L. 1995. Selecting multiproblem chemicals for risk reduction - a presentation of the Swedish Sunset Project. Solna, Sweden: Swedish National Chemicals Inspectorate (KEMI). ISSN:0284-1185

Gesellschaft für Strahlen-und Umweltforschung mbH, editor. 1986. Environmental modeling for priority setting among existing chemicals. Proceedings from a workshop 11–13 November 1985. Munich.

Klaassen CD, Eaton DL. 1993. Principles of toxicology. In: Amdur M, Doull J, Klaassen CD, editors. Casarett and Doull's toxicology: the basic science of poisons. 4th ed. New York NY: McGraw Hill.

Lewis Sr RJ, editor. 1992. Sax's dangerous properties of industrial materials. 8th ed. New York NY: Van Nostrand Reinhold.

McCarty LS, Mackay D. 1993. Enhancing ecolotoxicological modeling and assessment. *Environ Sci Technol* 27(9):1719–1728.

[OECD] Organization for Economic Cooperation and Development. 1986. Existing chemicals: systematic investigation, priority setting and chemicals reviews. Paris, France.

Samiullah Y. 1990. Prediction of the environmental fate of chemicals. New York NY: Elsevier Applied Science in association with the British Petroleum Company.

Swedish National Chemicals Inspectorate. 1995. Selecting multiproblem chemicals for risk reduction. In: Freij L, editor. Solna, Sweden: Swedish Sunset Project.

U.S. Congress, Office of Technology Assessment. September 1995. Screening and testing chemicals in commerce. Washington DC: Office of Technology Assessment. OTA-BP-ENV-166.

Workshop Participants

Karim Ahmed
Science and Policy Associates
Washington DC

Larry Barnthouse
Oak Ridge National Laboratory
Oak Ridge, Tennessee

Robert Boethling
U.S. Environmental Protection Agency
Washington DC

Richard Brown
Dow Chemical Company
Midland, Michigan

Rolf Bretz
Ciba-Geigy AG
Grenzach, Germany

Bernard Conilh de Beyassac
Environment Canada
Hull, Canada

Gary A. Davis
University of Tennessee
Knoxville, Tennessee

John Evans
Harvard University School of Public
    Health
Boston, Massachusetts

Franz Fiala
Austrian Standards Institute
Vienna, Austria

Dan Fort
U.S. Environmental Protection Agency
Washington DC

Emma Lou George
U.S. Environmental Protection Agency
Cincinnati, Ohio

John Giesy
Michigan State University
East Lansing, Michigan

Michael Gilbertson
Water Quality Board
International Joint Commission on the
    Great Lakes
Windsor, Ontario, Canada

James Gillett
Cornell University
Ithaca, New York

George Gray
Harvard University
Boston, Massachusetts

Bill Haaf
DuPont
Wilmington, Delaware

Bjørn Hansen
European Commission
Ispra, Italy

Rolf Hartung
University of Michigan
Ann Arbor, Michigan

Bill Hoffman
Motorola
Schaumburg, Illinois

Philip Howard
Syracuse Research Corporation
Syracuse, New York

Gary Hurlburt
Michigan Department of Natural
    Resources
Lansing, Michigan

Fran H. Irwin
World Resources Institute
Washington DC

David Jeffrey
EMCON
Sacramento, California

Allan Astrup Jensen
DK-Teknik
Soborg, Denmark

Jay Jon
U.S. Environmental Protection Agency
Washington DC

Sheila Jones
Directorate of Safety, Health and
  Environment
Aberdeen Proving Ground, Maryland

Baxter Jones
ICF Incorporated
Fairfax, Virginia

Ray Kent
U.S. Environmental Protection Agency
Washington DC

Yong-Hwa Kim
United Nations Industrial Development
  Organization
Vienna, Austria

Rich Kimerle
Monsanto Company
St. Louis, Missouri

Preben Kristensen
Water Quality Institute
Harsholm, Denmark

Robert Larson
The Proctor & Gamble Company
Cincinnati, Ohio

Lynne Fahey McGrath
Hoechst Celanese Corporation
Somerville, New Jersey

Kathy Monk
U.S. Environmental Protection Agency
Washington DC

Ron Newhook
Health Canada
Ottawa, Ontario, Canada

Heinz-Jochen Poremski
Umweltbundesamt
Berlin, Germany

Richard Purdy
3M Company
St. Paul, Minnesota

Mark Ralston
U.S. Environmental Protection Agency
Washington DC

Kevin Reinert
Rohm and Haas Company
Spring House, Pennsylvania

Rosalind Rolland
World Wildlife Fund
Washington DC

Robert Ross
Oak Ridge National Laboratory
Oak Ridge, Tennessee

Friedrich Schmidt-Bleek
Wuppertal Institute for Climate,
  Environment & Energy
North Rhine-Westphalia, Wuppertal,
Germany

Adam Socha
Ontario Ministry of Environment and
  Energy
Toronto, Ontario, Canada

Mike Stevens
Monsanto Company
St. Louis, Missouri

Bradford Strohm
General Motors
Detroit, Michigan

Mary Swanson
University of Tennessee
Knoxville, Tennessee

Duane Tolle
Battelle Columbus Division
Columbus, Ohio

Pauline Wagner
U.S. Environmental Protection Agency
Washington DC

John Walker
U.S. Environmental Protection Agency
Washington DC

Bob Wilson
Landbank Environmental
London, United Kingdom

Maurice Zeeman
U.S. Environmental Protection Agency
Washington DC

Sources of Data for Chemical Ranking and Scoring Purposes

A number of databases provided by several vendors are convenient sources of information suitable for chemical ranking and scoring purposes. Nonbibliographic ("factual") databases provide endpoint values such as NOAELs and LD50s, bioconcentration factors, and short descriptions of the corresponding studies. These types of databases can be exceptionally good secondary sources of information. Those such as AQUIRE are peer reviewed, with study reliability indicators assigned to their records. Bibliographic databases provide the user with references to specific research papers and books for follow-up, although some also provide abstracts, e.g. the versions of *Chemical Abstracts* (CA SEARCH) and *Biological Abstracts* (BIOSIS) provided in North America by Science and Technical Network (STN) International.

The following is a brief guide to some readily available on-line and/or on-disk databases.

U.S. National Library of Medicine (MEDLARS, TOXNET)

The Toxicology Data Network (TOXNET) is a component of the U.S. National Library of Medicine's Medical Literature Access and Retrieval System (MEDLARS) on-line information system. TOXNET contains five files of toxicological information: Chemical Carcinogenesis Information System (CCRIS), Genotoxicity Database (GENETOX), Hazardous Substances Databank (HSDB), NIOSH's Registry of Toxic Effects of Chemical Substances (RTECS) and USEPA's Integrated Risk Information System (IRIS). The latter is a database containing dose-response assessment information, USEPA carcinogenicity classifications, and USEPA regulatory information for over 250 chemical substances. IRIS is updated on a regular basis, and as such it is a good source of current U.S. environmental regulatory information for specific substances.

Another component of MEDLARS, the E.L. Hill (ELHILL) system, contains bibliographic files on medicine and clinical studies which may be useful: Medical Information On-line (MEDLINE), Toxicology Information On-line (TOXLINE), and Cancer Literature database (CANCERLIT).

Canadian Centre for Occupational Health and Safety Information System

The Canadian Centre for Occupational Health and Safety Information System (CCINFO) is an information retrieval system provided on-line and on CD-ROM by the Canadian Centre for Occupational Health and Safety (CCOHS). Several bibliographic and nonbibliographic databases contain occupational health and safety information on specific substances as well as information on Canadian occupational health and pesticide regulations. Many of CCINFO's databases are available in both English and French.

Some pertinent CCINFO databases are Material Safety Data Sheets (MSDSs) for trade-name products; RTECS, the U.S. NIOSH's toxicity information database; Chemical Evaluation Search and Retrieval System (CESARS), a database containing use, fate, and toxicity information on chemicals found or used in the Great Lakes Basin, produced by the Michigan Department of Natural Resources (MDNR) and the Ontario Ministry of Environment and Energy (OMOEE); Canadian Regulatory Information on Pesticide Products (RIPP); substance-specific occupational health and safety summaries from CCOHS (Chemical Information [CHEMINFO] database) and from the New Jersey Department of Health Services; various files on specific occupational health and safety topics including noise levels, health effects of nickel compounds, and radiation exposure.

USEPA MED Ecotoxicology Data Systems

The United States Environmental Protection Agency's Mid-Continent Ecology Division (MED) in Duluth, Minnesota, provides four databases to government users. Some are available to the public through commercial vendors such as Chemical Information System (CIS).

QSAR (quantitative structure-activity relationship) is a modeling system that provides estimates of physical–chemical properties, environmental fate, and toxic effects of substances through the application of several models derived from molecular structure analysis. QSAR can be used to identify high-risk substances when experimental (laboratory or field) data are unavailable. For a substance of interest, the user enters its Chemical Abstracts Service (CAS) Registry number or Simplified Molecular Line Input System (SMILES) format line-notation structure description, and where possible the system will use appropriate QSAR models to generate estimated values.

AQUIRE (Aquatic Toxicity Information Retrieval Database) provides a comprehensive compilation of aquatic toxicity test results including acute, sublethal, and bioaccumulation information for individual substances, culled from published scientific reports. Test species include freshwater and saltwater animals and plants, with the exception of aquatic birds, adult amphibians, mammals, and bacteria other than blue-green algae. AQUIRE contains the results of over 129,000 toxicity tests from 9,000 references for over 5,600 substances and 2,827 aquatic species. The database was last updated in 1994.

ASTER (ASsessment Tools for the Evaluation of Risk) consolidates key toxicology information from the AQUIRE and QSAR databases that is useful for risk assessment.

ECOTOX (Ecotoxicology database) is the newest system, comprising the MED's AQUIRE database as well as two databases developed by the USEPA's Western Ecology Division (WED), PHYTOTOX for phytotoxicology information (see below) and TERRETOX for terrestrial wildlife toxicology information. The USEPA Office of Pesticide Programs Ecological Effects Branch's Ecological Effects DataBase (EEDB) of the ecological effects of pesticides will be included in ECOTOX in the near future.

PHYTOTOX

The phytoxicology database PHYTOTOX was developed by the USEPA WED environmental research laboratory in Corvallis, Oregon and the University of Oklahoma. It is available on diskettes or on-line. PHYTOTOX contains information on the effects of over 2,000 organic substances on 1,300 terrestrial plant species, represented by over 74,000 toxicity tests from 3,900 references through the year 1987.

Risk Reduction Engineering Laboratory

The USEPA Risk Reduction Engineering Laboratory (RREL) Treatability Database (USEPA 1994c) is a good source of information related to the treatment of wastewater, including degradation and removal data for substances in wastewater.

International Registry of Potentially Toxic Chemicals

The International Registry of Potentially Toxic Chemicals (IRPTC) is provided by the United Nations Environment Programme and made available through government agencies of various nations. IRPTC aims to provide its users with information necessary to assess the risk presented by chemicals to humans and the environment.

To facilitate management of information, the version of IRPTC provided through the Canadian Department of National Health has been divided into several sub-files. The *IRPTC Legal* file contains international recommendations and regulatory information related to the control of chemical substances in media such as air, water, wastes, soil, sediments, animal and plant tissues, food, drugs, and consumer products. The *Chemiobiokinetics* file contains information on the absorption, distribution, metabolism, and excretion of drugs, chemicals, and metabolites. The *Mammalian Toxicity and Special Toxicity Studies* files contain information on the toxic effects of chemicals on laboratory and domestic mammals. Additional substance-specific information can be found in the *IRPTC Identifiers, Production, Processes and Waste (IPPW), Environmental Fate Tests*, and *Environmental Fate and Pathways into the Environment* files.

Pesticide Research Information System

Agriculture Canada's Pesticide Research Information System (PRIS) provides information on the development of pesticides and biocontrol agents from research and development to registration in Canada. Included is information on experimental pesticides research, residues data, regulatory information and a use index.

National Pesticide Information Retrieval System

The National Pesticide Information Retrieval System (NPIRS) contains information about pesticides registered in the United States, including product information, Material Safety Data Sheets (MSDSs) and USEPA Fact Sheets. The latter provide chemical, environmental, and toxicological information, descriptions of the active substances, use patterns, regulatory information, and corresponding rationale.

STN International

STN International is a database vendor specializing in the fields of pure and applied chemistry, physics and biological sciences. Files of particular interest include *Chemical Abstracts* (CA SEARCH), *Chemical Abstracts Service Registry* (REGISTRY), *Biological Abstracts* (BIOSIS) and *National Technical Information Service* (NTIS). CA SEARCH contains bibliographic references and abstracts of papers covering all properties of chemical substances including toxic effects. BIOSIS is similar but concentrates on comprehensive coverage of the life sciences. REGISTRY is an index file of chemical names, useful for finding CAS registry numbers, primary substance names as per the American Chemical Society's CAS 9th Collective Index, synonyms, molecular formulas, and structural diagrams for specific substances. NTIS contains references to and abstracts of technical reports sponsored by the U.S. federal government.

DIALOG Information Services

DIALOG encompasses several hundred databases covering an exceptionally wide variety of topics. They provide mainly bibliographic reference information although some directories and factual databases are available.

Of particular relevance to chemical ranking and scoring are CA SEARCH, BIOSIS, and NTIS (see above under STN), as well as *Science Citation Index* (SCISEARCH), a multidisciplinary bibliographic index of literature in the fields of science and technology, pure and applied.

Chemical Information System

Chemical Information System (CIS) is an integrated on-line database system covering several subjects related to chemistry. Available database files provide data such as chemical identifiers, physical–chemical properties, toxicity, environmental effects, analytical data, and U.S. regulatory status information. Many of the databases on CIS were originally developed by the USEPA.

Of particular interest are Oil and Hazardous Materials/Technical Assistance Data System (OHM/TACS), which contains extensive information on oils and hazardous materials; Information System for Hazardous Organics in Water (ISHOW), which contains physical data; Structure and Nomenclature Search System (SANSS), a system for identifying chemicals by name and structure; and Toxic Substances Control Act Plant and Production Search System (TSCAPP), which contains production data for 55,000 chemicals named under the U.S. Toxic Substances Control Act (TSCA). CIS also is the commercial vendor for the U.S. government databases AQUIRE, CESARS, GENETOX, IRIS, PHYTOTOX, and RTECS mentioned elsewhere in this appendix.

The CIS Environmental Fate (ENVIROFATE) database contains environmental fate information. It is essentially the same as the Chemical Fate (CHEMFATE) database available through the NTIS, although it is generally not as up-to-date as CHEMFATE.

Syracuse Research Corporation

The Syracuse Research Corporation's (SRC) database system contains bibliographic and nonbibliographic information on the environmental fate, biodegradation and persistence of many chemical substances, in its Environmental Fate Database (EFDB), including CHEMFATE subfile, BIOLOG, BIODEG, and DATALOG databases. SRC also includes Physical Properties database (PHYSPROP), a source of basic physical–chemical properties data and Toxic Substances Control Act Test Submissions (TSCATS), a large database of unpublished technical data submitted to the USEPA by industry under the TSCA. TSCATS includes health, environmental fate, and environmental effects study results.

International Uniform Chemical Information Database

The International Uniform Chemical Information Database (IUCLID) is Oracle-based and is a multilingual (currently the original nine European Union [EU] languages), glossary-based database that contains the data on the EU high production volume chemicals, which has been submitted by industry following Council Regulation EEC/793/93. The IUCLID database software is copyrighted by the European Commission and is available through the ECB at cost recovery for the installation. The IUCLID has been or is being installed at the 15 EU Member States (with multiple installations in some Member States), approximately 40 European companies, the Organization for Economic Cooperation and Development (OECD) secretariat in Paris, the IRPTC in Geneva, the USEPA in Washington, and Japan. The major part of this data is nonconfidential, including the physical–chemical properties, chemical fate and pathways, ecotoxicity and toxicity data. The nonconfidential data are available on a CD either as an IUCLID export file (readable only by IUCLID software) or as a low-cost, stand-alone, simple database.

Table B1 Index to pertinent environmental toxicology databases

Topic area	Database mnemonic and system
Bioaccumulation and bioconcentration	AQUIRE (USEPA MED, CIS) ASTER, ECOTOX (USEPA MED) CESARS (CCINFO, CIS) HSDB (TOXNET)
Chemical, physical, environmental fate, and biodegradation properties	BIODEG (SRC) CESARS (CCINFO, CIS) CHEMFATE, PHYSPROP (SRC) ENVIROFATE (CIS) HEILBRON (DIALOG) ISHOW (CIS) MERCK (DIALOG, CIS) OHM/TADS (CIS) RREL Treatability Database (USEPA RREL)
Production and emission volumes	CESARS (CCINFO, CIS) Toxics Release Inventory (TRI) (TOXNET) TSCAPP (CIS)
General toxicology	BIOSIS (STN, DIALOG) CA SEARCH (STN, DIALOG) CCRIS (TOXNET, CIS) CESARS (CCINFO, CIS) Excerpta Medica database (EMBASE) (DIALOG) HSDB (TOXNET) OHM/TADS (CIS) Merck (CIS, DIALOG) RTECS (CCINFO, TOXNET, DIALOG, CIS) TSCATS (CIS, SRC)
Genotoxicity	GENETOX (TOXNET, CIS)
Reproductive toxicology	Developmental and Reproductive Toxicity (DART) (TOXNET)
Aquatic and environmental toxicology	AQUIRE (USEPA MED, CIS) Aquatic Science and Fisheries Abstracts (ASFA) (DIALOG) ASTER, ECOTOX (USEPA MED)
Phytotoxicology	PHYTOMED (STN) PHYTOTOX (USEPA WED, CIS) ECOTOX (USEPA MED)
Regulatory information	CHEMINFO (CCINFO) Chemical Regulations and Guidelines System (CRGS) (DIALOG) IRIS (TOXNET, CIS) IRPTC (United Nations Environment Programme) RIPP (CCINFO) RTECS (CCINFO, TOXNET, DIALOG, CIS)

SETAC

A Professional Society for Environmental Scientists and Engineers and Related Disciplines Concerned with Environmental Quality

The Society of Environmental Toxicology and Chemistry (SETAC), with offices in North America and Europe, is a nonprofit, professional society that provides a forum for individuals and institutions engaged in the study of environmental problems, management and regulation of natural resources, education, research and development, and manufacturing and distribution.

Goals

- Promote research, education, and training in the environmental sciences
- Promote systematic application of all relevant scientific disciplines to the evaluation of chemical hazards
- Participate in scientific interpretation of issues concerned with hazard assessment and risk analysis
- Support development of ecologically acceptable practices and principles
- Provide a forum for communication among professionals in government, business, academia, and other segments of society involved in the use, protection, and management of our environment

Activities

- Annual meetings with study and workshop sessions, platform and poster papers, and achievement and merit awards
- Monthly scientific journal, *Environmental Toxicology and Chemistry*, SETAC newsletter, and special technical publications
- Funds for education and training through the SETAC Scholarship/Fellowship Program
- Chapter forums for the presentation of scientific data and for the interchange and study of information about local concerns
- Advice and counsel to technical and nontechnical persons through a number of standing and *ad hoc* committees

Membership

SETAC's growing membership includes more than 5,000 individuals from government, academia, business, and public-interest groups with technical backgrounds in chemistry, toxicology, biology, ecology, atmospheric sciences, health sciences, earth sciences, and engineering.

If you have training in these or related disciplines and are engaged in the study, use, or management of environmental resources, SETAC can fulfill your professional affiliation needs. Membership categories include Associate, Student, Senior Active, and Emeritus.

For more information, contact SETAC, 1010 North 12th Avenue, Pensacola, Florida 32501-3370; T 850 469 1500; F 850 469 9778; E setac@setac.org; http://www.setac.org.